Dentist on the Ward

12th Edition

An Introduction to Oral and Maxillofacial Surgery and Medicine for Core Trainees in Dentistry

Andrew Sadler and Leo Cheng

Dentist on the Ward

Preface to 12th Edition

For this 12th edition, all chapters have been re-edited, most shortened, and some updated to reflect developing priorities in oral and maxillofacial surgery and hospital healthcare.

Dentist on the Ward provides:

1. An introduction to the hospital and essential information necessary for the new dentally qualified trainee in oral and maxillofacial surgery.

2. Advice on surgery from preparing the patient for operation to post-operative care and complications.

3. Urgent care, including being on call for the emergency department. The situations and clinical conditions the dental core trainee is likely to have to deal with, including diagnosis of facial trauma. The initial management of medical emergencies that might be encountered is explained.

4. Background and introduction to the practical skills that a dental core trainee may need to gain in their job.

5. Medical topics which are most relevant to surgery and particularly oral and maxillofacial surgery.

6. An introduction to the clinical work of oral and maxillofacial surgeons. The chapters should help the understanding of the rationale behind the surgery and the routine oral medicine and pathology cases that present to oral and maxillofacial surgeons. These chapters are succinct for easy reading in a short time. However, we believe they cover the essential elements required for examination candidates at undergraduate and general postgraduate examinations in dentistry.

The book should help the dental trainee engage with their work and provide the most relevant background information to get the most out of it. However, the most valuable learning, as in any clinical subject, is practical experience, seeing and participating in treating patients and discussing the cases with colleagues. This book should be a good prequel to that.

Andrew Sadler and Leo Cheng January 2022

First Edition Published   2010
12th Edition 2022

ISBN: 978-1-9993612-6-6

Dentist on the Ward

Contents

Introduction

Surgery

Urgent Care

Practical Skills

Most Relevant Medical Topics

Introduction to Conditions Managed in OMFS

1. <u>Why work in Oral and Maxillofacial Surgery?</u>

Most of the work coming into oral and maxillofacial departments (OMFS) is of direct relevance to dentistry. This work provides a wealth of potential learning material for the recently qualified dental surgeon; this includes oral medicine, temporomandibular joint problems, facial pain, benign oral swellings, surgery complementary to orthodontics as well as dento-alveolar surgery, and dental extraction work on medically compromised patients.

The most beneficial time to take a junior post in OMFS is about a year after qualifying. You will have developed some considerable skill in the handling of anxious patients, some considerable dexterity in carrying out operative procedures, and an understanding of dentistry within the primary care sector; this will be of help in understanding the problems of those who refer patients into the hospital. You may pass on some of this benefit to your senior colleagues who have not worked in primary care dentistry for many years, if at all.

The main reason to take a job will remain the opportunity to learn, but you can also expect it to be fun. It may be the first time that you are working as part of a team managing individual patients. Team working can be enjoyable, especially in times of difficulty, and the camaraderie and sense of common purpose gives added enjoyment to the work. It is probable that, at least at the beginning, you will discuss almost every patient you see with another colleague, which is unlikely to be the case in a primary dental practice.

At the end of one year in an OMFS department, we would usually recommend moving on rather than staying longer in the same department. If you are intending to work elsewhere within dentistry, you have probably got as much out of the speciality as you are going to and if you intend to have a career in OMFS, then it will probably be better in the long term to complement your experience elsewhere.

At the end of a one year post in OMFS, aim to be competent at performing most dental extractions (surgical or otherwise), the initial management of dental trauma, interpretation of dental radiographs and facial X-rays and CT scans. You should have seen most common oral mucosal conditions, some maxillofacial prosthetics and implantology, patients with chronic facial pain and some orthognathic surgery. In some

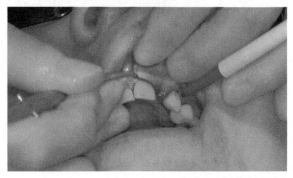

You should be able to treat most dento-alveolar conditions.

units, you may have seen patients with cleft lip and palate and other developmental anomalies. You will hopefully understand temporo-mandibular joint disorders, outpatient management of patients with common co-existing medical problems, working relationships with other disciplines such as orthodontics, restorative dentistry and ENT surgery and the issues regarding general anaesthesia and conscious sedation. You should also understand clinical governance and have taken part in clinical audit.

The best way to study for postgraduate examinations is to read around and discuss clinical

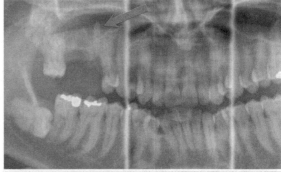

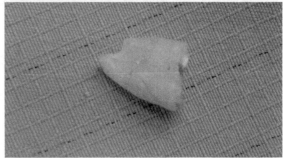

You will learn the management of complications such as this root displaced into the maxillary antrum.

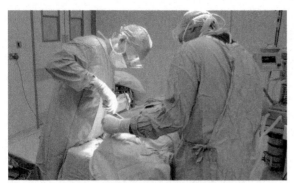

You can learn to work as part of a team and operate on simple trauma and dento-alveolar conditions as well as assisting in major cases.

cases and you should have seen plenty of clinical material to help you with post graduate clinical examinations. Studying for examinations while working encourages a discipline of approach and makes the daily clinical tasks more interesting. Writing about and presenting interesting clinical cases is a skill well worth cultivating and will enrich your subsequent clinical career.

In applying for jobs, be aware that there are still many units which provide inferior jobs for their junior trainees, or where it may simply be not very pleasant to work. If you can, try to work in a single site unit. Avoid jobs where you will be expected to drive between different hospitals, or where you might have to work in a hospital peripheral to the main unit when there is no one senior present to advise or help you. Be wary of jobs where there are many house surgeons working shifts to cover busy trauma commitments at night.

Check that there is sufficient clinical work in the department for the number of trainees and that when carrying out minor oral surgery, there is adequate support, supervision and teaching. You can do this by speaking to the present incumbents. Always ask direct questions and talk to more than one to get a balanced picture; be wary of over enthusiastic reports as some young people can be uncritical and sycophantic to their seniors beyond justification. Give an especially wide berth to departments where the trainees run errands or get little supervised operating experience. You may find that practical surgical experience is given preferentially to second or third year dental core trainees and those in the first year get little or none. If this is the situation, you may want to walk away and apply to a smaller unit. Practical operating experience is the foundation of learning surgery; if the trainees don't get enough supervised operating to do, don't work there.

We asked some core dental trainees what they learned in working in OMFS. This is what they told us:

Working in a team.

Developed presentation skills.

Got involved in a research project.

Became a more rounded clinician.

Developed patient and medical management skills.

Worked in a department with other young like-minded clinicians.

Appreciated the systemic health of patients as well as their dentition.

Learnt to work in stressful situations.

Leaned to deal with patients who were frightened or under the influence of drugs or alcohol.

Improved time management and priorities when faced with several problems.

Developed confidence with multiple medical problems.

Had hands on practice at minor oral surgery.

Saw patients presenting with oral cancer and pre-cancerous conditions.

Initially managed patients with sepsis and drained abscesses.

Saw orthognathic surgery before a career in orthodontics.

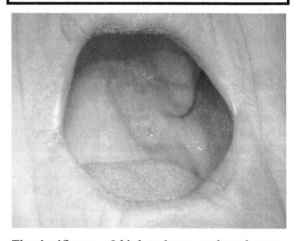

The significance of this lymphoma on the palate was missed by the dentist who eased the patient's denture away from it. An OMFS department is the best place to become familiar with dangerous oral conditions.

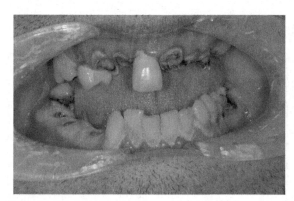

You should be able to carry out a lot of surgical extractions.

Students

Several universities arrange for their dental students to have attachments to OMFS departments. We believe that the experience gained from such an attachment is well worthwhile and will be enhanced by a little thought and planning before starting, as well as a proactive attitude on arrival. Our experience is that surgeons are usually keen to have students in their departments and specialist registrars and core trainees are often very willing to help and teach them.

For students, our advice is to go with a 'shopping list' of types of clinical cases you wish to see. Take histories from the patients (ask if you can), examine them, look up what investigations have been done, see the results, ask questions and read around the cases. Ideally, present the cases to someone such as a consultant or specialist registrar and provoke a discussion on the management of the patient from which you can learn. It is best to choose cases which will be of use to you to prepare for your examinations or practice of dentistry.

List of priority things to do on student elective

Hands on practice at exodontia & minor oral surgery if possible, particularly if there are dental extractions under general anaesthetic

See patients presenting with oral cancer. Listen to the history, examine & palpate the lesion & lymphatic drainage, follow the investigation & find out what the treatment is to be

Get experience in venepuncture; particularly ask the anaesthetist to teach you in theatre

Take a full history from a patient with an oral medical condition, see several with white patches in the mouth & learn which ones might be pre-cancerous & which ones you would refer if you were working in dental practice

Take a history from a patient with post extraction haemorrhage, note their management & what tests and observations are done & why. See a patient with post extraction osteitis

Take a history and examine a patient with a severe dental abscess; note their investigation and management

See a patient with a fractured mandible, particularly observe the management of dental injuries & use this as a basis for learning current management of dental trauma

Observe hospital cross infection control

See some orthognathic surgery; you must see the patient before and after the surgery to appreciate the problem. (Do this for all patients whose surgery you observe if possible.)

See a major cancer operation but don't waste all day observing one case unless you get some suturing practice

2. <u>Education and Health. Patient Confidentiality</u>

There are several matters which will need to be considered before starting a hospital job in oral and maxillofacial surgery or which you should know about from the beginning. You will be sent essential information by your employer and speaking to one of several of those working in the department before you can also be invaluable.

Occupational Health

Before starting clinical work in a hospital, you will need a health assessment, which will start with a communicable disease questionnaire. This is may be carried out by a nurse or done on-line. You will need a history of your immunisation and blood tests for hepatitis B titre level, hepatitis B antigen, hepatitis C antibody, HIV antibody, measles antibody, rubella antibody and chickenpox antibody. An appointment will be arranged for you to see an occupational health nurse. You will be examined to check if you have a scar from BCG immunisation and, if not, a T-Spot test will be carried out. Additional blood tests will be carried out if required for the above diseases, and if a problem is identified, an appointment made to see an occupational health physician. This will normally take place as soon as you start work; you may not be able see patients until you have been 'cleared'.

Health care workers who are HIV positive may now carry out exposure-prone procedures, provided they are taking effective anti-retroviral drug therapy and if they have an undetectable viral load and are monitored by an occupational health physician. Self-testing kits are now available for HIV.

Each autumn, all staff in contact with patients will be offered immunisation against the current strains of influenza. This is usually carried out in the workplace by nurses who prowl the hospital looking for recipients.

Education and appraisal

You will probably be involved in an appraisal process where you can discuss your experience and progress in the job. This will probably be three times in a year and will normally be conducted with your 'educational supervisor, who is most likely to be one of your consultants. They should act as a mentor, giving guidance and feedback about your performance and pastoral support. The first appraisal will probably

---

> *<u>Example of Personal Development Plan</u>*
>
> 1. Gain more confidence in diagnosis and management of white patches in the mouth
>
> 2. Remove more impacted third molars. Target : 20 cases by April
>
> 3. Finish audit project by May
>
> 4. Pass postgraduate examination by June
>
> *The goals should follow the principle of SMART: Specific, Measurable, Achievable, Realistic and Timed.*

be within a few weeks of your starting and the last just before you finish. Appraisals are a two-way process and you should be able to feedback if your clinical work experience is inadequate to meet your reasonable learning objectives.

At the first appraisal, you should discuss your Personal Development Plan. This should be a short list of the goals you wish to achieve. The most popular and possibly the most useful goal is practical experience in minor surgery. Keep a log of the number of cases you have performed and assisted at. This is useful in assessing whether you are getting sufficient practical experience, and for the educational supervisor to feed back to colleagues to ensure you get adequate experience.

You should keep a 'portfolio'. This will normally be in electronic form (e-portfolio). It should contain a record of work-based assessments, any projects or audits in progress, multi-source feedback, a log of your activity, and progress in examinations. You should keep records of all training events you have attended within your place of work and elsewhere, and your reflections of any benefit gained. The portfolio can evidence when applying for future jobs and for any validation required by any regulatory body.

We would recommend that you use your clinical experience to prepare yourself for postgraduate examinations. Studying for post-graduate examinations and qualifications provides a goal to aim for and encourages reading around clinical work, which makes it more enjoyable as well as facilitating career progression.

Besides improving your clinical skills, you should also consider other skills which may be useful in your subsequent career, such as presenting cases, writing, improving your skills in using software and, if the opportunity arises, by teaching experience with dental/nursing students.

Your employing NHS Trust will insist that you receive some statutory (required by law) and mandatory (required by employer) training in various core topics. Mandatory training may take many forms, particularly on-line learning programmes on your employer's intranet and attendance at specific training sessions during working hours. Remember to keep records of all meetings, training, and certificates in your portfolio.

Confidentiality

There are many ways in which confidentiality can be breached in a hospital, which are unlikely to occur in a dental practice. You will work as a team, which involves discussing patients with colleagues, accessing computer based patients' records, photographing and discussing cases at clinical meetings and contact with relatives.

This topic will probably form one module of the mandatory training. Below we have listed some dos and don'ts which from our experience can lead to problems.

Advice from previous trainees

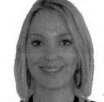

Sara

'Never be worried about asking for help. If you are ever unsure, it is always better to ask. Work hard and be prepared to study alongside to ensure you get a lot out of it.'

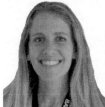

Julia

'You've got to be proactive and say I'm really interested in this case; can I do this? I really want to learn. I have noticed that if, for example, if there's an ectopic canine and we've got an expose and bond I'm interested in that and I say please can I raise the flap, please can I do that they are so supportive and they want you to learn and they are impressed that you say 'I want to do this'.

Protecting confidentiality

<u>Do</u>

Discard anything written about patients only in secure rubbish bins for shredding

Log out of the hospital computer system when you have finished looking at patients' records

Make sure you are following hospital policy when taking clinical photographs

Use a hospital encrypted memory stick for any patient related information

Email on the secure NHS system anything relating to patients (e.g. nhs.net)

Only discuss patients with their relatives if you are sure they have consented

Keep your password to the hospital computer system secure

<u>Do Not</u>

Discuss patients where you can be overheard

Leave notes or patient records where they can be seen by someone not involved with their care

Discuss patients out of the work environment

Gossip about patients you know personally or who are famous

Take photographs on personal cameras or mobile phones

Show clinical photographs out of the clinical environment

Access clinical records of any person whose care you are not involved with

---

Have objectives of what you want to get, write them down and make a personal development plan with targets for them such as by January done ? cases of X. Speak to people and use that opportunity to speak to other disciplines such as paediatrics, orthodontics and medical consultants. Get advice for if you're not sure what you want to do you can get advice on all sorts of different things and you can get to see what you enjoy and what you don't enjoy.'

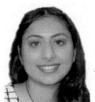

Preeya

'I think there is a lot of anxiety around starting an OMFS job particularly because it is quite different to anything we have experienced. I think many people are just getting over the anxt of it and putting a lot of pressure on themselves but I think the main thing that the whole of the Max Fax team in the hospital they are

aware that you've never done an OMFS job before. They're there to support you so if you have any issues the main thing is to try not to stress and to do things on your own. The most important thing is to ask for help because you will be in scenarios where you are a vital team member and it is a scenario where a patient can be very unwell which is very different from a patient getting dental pain. The best thing is to approach a senior member and make sure you get a clear history from the patient, try to formulate the best history, medical history, social history so that you can transfer that information on and then get the help you need.'

Ohsun

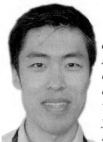

'Never be afraid to ask questions no matter how simple or stupid they sound, because at the end of the day we're there to look after the patient. A second thing is when you are on call for Max Fax you sometimes have lots of jobs scattered all around the hospital. I try to do them in blocks and try to ensure that I do the easier ones first; but it's always complicated because you always must prioritise emergencies that are coming along. So there are a lot of things to learn and you have to reflect each day to see where you can make improvements.'

Sanford

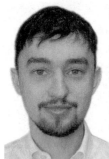

'I would agree, ask lots of questions, especially early on whenever you're in theatre or clinics and you see something you don't understand. You're surrounded by highly skilled clinicians and should take advantage of the opportunity to learn as much as possible. Also make the most of the year by getting involved with projects. Take opportunities you may not necessarily have in practice or other environments.'

Sanaa

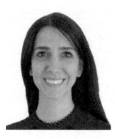

'I agree it's all really about being focused and organised.

But I think you do have to get out of it what you want. You can't start a job assuming it's all going to be given to you and

as a Max Fax trainee I think you have to be proactive. You could easily sit in theatre and not be involved because the consultant surgeons are focused on the patient and not you but if you show some interest and give things a go then ultimately you get back what you put in.'

Example of Topics to Discuss at first Appraisal

1. Previous experience in last job

2. Accommodation arrangements

3. Problems encountered so far

4. Thoughts on future career

5. Aspirations for the job

6. Audit project

7. Postgraduate examinations

---

3. <u>Hospital Cross Infection Control</u>

Methicillin Resistant Staphylococcus Aureus (MRSA)

Staphylococcus aureus is common in air, clothing, bedding and dust, where it can survive for several weeks. It is also carried by approximately 40% of healthy adults in their noses and, to a lesser extent, in their throats and faeces. It can develop resistance to antibiotics by adaptation and can flourish at the expense of antibiotic sensitive organisms.

The most commonly used antibiotic for treating staph. aureus infection was flucloxacillin; when the organism is resistant to flucloxacillin, it is known as MRSA (Methicillin Resistant Staphylococcus Aureus). This is because the older drug methicillin is used to test sensitivity because in vitro it accurately mimics the in vivo behaviour of flucloxacillin. In fact, oxycycline is commonly used for testing nowadays, but it is still known as MRSA. MRSA has been known, and been increasing in prevalence, since the 1960s.

MRSA and other drug-resistant bacteria exist because of over-use of antibiotics. Patients and others can be 'colonised' by MRSA with no pathogenic response. They are said to have become 'infected' when the patient develops inflammatory signs or symptoms. The greatest risk of MRSA is in those patients who have surgical wounds, are immunocompromised or have serious debilitating illness. It is of low risk to those in outpatient clinics, paediatric or general medical wards, but the risk will be greater in the intensive care, oncology and renal wards.

The mainstay of prevention of colonisation and infection of patients with MRSA is a high standard of routine cross infection control, such as hand washing, using protective clothing, good cleaning and isolation of colonised or infected patients.

Those who are admitted to a surgical ward are normally screened by taking swabs for culture from their hairline, nostrils, axillae, groin and any wounds. A patient found to be infected or colonised is 'barrier nursed' in a single room. The room should be maintained clean and contain no unnecessary furniture. Staff entering should wear gloves and aprons, which should be disposed of on leaving the room. Staff should enter only when necessary; wounds should be covered and strict hand hygiene should be observed.

Patients colonised by MRSA may be decolonised by using mupirocin 2% ointment to the nostrils three

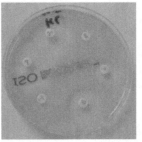 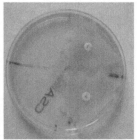

Staphylococcus aureus on agar plate. Sensitivity is indicated by the inhibition of growth by antibiotics discs.

MRSA. Growth is uninhibited by the Oxycycline discs.

times a day; antiseptic detergent should be used for a total body bath or shower, which should include the hair; colonised wounds should be treated with povidone-iodine. If staff are found to be colonised, then an attempt should be made to reverse this with mupirocin. If working in high-risk areas such as intensive care or the renal unit, then they may have to cease work temporarily until decontaminated and have had three consecutive negative swabs from hairline, nostrils, axillae and groin.

Clostridium Difficile (C.diff)

Clostridium difficile, commonly referred to as C. diff., is an anaerobic bacterium which lives harmlessly in the gut of approximately 3% of the normal population. It is usually kept in check by other commensal gut organisms, but if these are reduced by broad-spectrum antibiotics, then C. diff. can propagate in large amounts, releasing Toxin A and Toxin B which can damage the gut wall leading to ulceration, bleeding and diarrhoea. The diarrhoea can vary from being brief and self-limiting to a severe pseudo-membranous colitis with gut perforation and death. Those who are most at risk of the severest disease are the elderly with serious co-existing disease.

Although 3% of adults carry it in their guts, most cases of C. diff. diarrhoea arise from cross infection from others who have excreted spores in their faeces, which have been ingested. The spores are resistant to alcohol.

The main action we can take to reduce this disease is to be judicious in using broad-spectrum antibiotics. Antibiotics should be used only when absolutely necessary. In our hospitals, there is a policy governing their use for certain conditions and they are automatically stopped after five days. Certain broad-spectrum antibiotics can only be prescribed with the permission of a consultant microbiologist. Secondly, patients who have C. diff. should be isolated and barrier nursed and thirdly we should be meticulous about hand hygiene on the wards and if there is a patient around who has diarrhoea, then hands should be washed with soap and water rather than using alcoholic hand rub, as the spores are alcohol resistant.

When carrying out procedures on patients, you should wear personal protective equipment (PPE); apron, mask, goggles and gloves. Such procedures include changing dressings or IV lines on the ward or cannulating patients. There is no evidence to show that anything more is necessary when carrying out minor surgery, such as dental extraction or biopsy, in the outpatient facility. However, the house rules or custom may be to wear a full theatre gown for these procedures, in which case you should abide by them.

Hand Hygiene

Good hand hygiene is probably the single most important method of combatting cross infection. You will find there are many hand wash basins with soap and taps that can be controlled with elbows, available in all clinical areas of the hospital. Hands should be washed before and after starting work, after using the toilet, before eating, and when the hands are obviously contaminated.

In addition to this, the hands must be cleaned with an alcohol rub on entering or leaving a ward or clinical area, in between seeing patients and before carrying out an aseptic procedure. Containers with alcohol rub will be available at all hand basins and at the entrance to and within all clinical areas as well at the end of beds on the wards. The alcohol rub should only be used on

visibly clean hands; otherwise, they should be washed with soap and water beforehand. Hand cream will also be available in ward areas and should be used after high frequency of hand washing, before breaks and at the end of work.

Covid 19

The Covid 19 pandemic has caused a delay in surgery for other patients and a tremendous increase in the number of patients waiting for treatment.

As the virus mutates and changes its personality, the challenges will continue to change and each hospital will be keenly following the best evidence on how to adapt, and you can expect guidance to change significantly over time.

You will inevitably be given details of the policy being followed at the time when undergoing induction for your new job and you will be expected to follow these policies, be immunised and take care.

Putting on Personal Protective Equipment (PPE) (apron, mask, goggles and gloves)

PPE should be worn to reduce the chance of you spreading infection from one patient to another and for your own protection. It should be used when carrying out procedures on patients which involve contact with saliva, blood or when attending to any open wound. It should also be worn when entering a room where a patient is being nursed in isolation because they have an infection. You should pay attention to putting on your PPE and taking it off in the correct order.

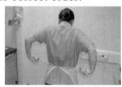

1. After washing hands put on apron- place over head and tie at back

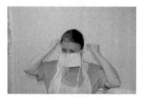

2. Put on mask ensuring a good seal between mask and face.

3. Put on goggles

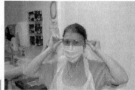

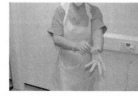

4. Put on gloves

Hand cleaning: use the same hand movements when washing or using alcohol solution Should only take 15 to 30 seconds

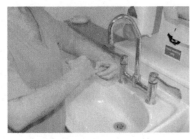

1. Take off rings and watches and ensure bare below elbows.

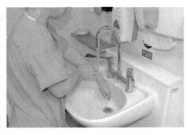

2. Turn on taps and wet hands thoroughly.

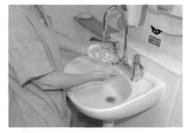

3. Generous soap application, enough to cover hands completely.

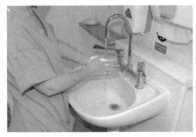

4. Rub palms together to generate a good lather.

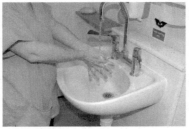

5. Rub palm onto back of hand with fingers interlocked.

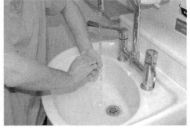

6. Cup hands together to clean back of fingers and nails.

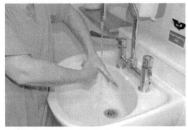

7. Scrub thumbs with a twisting motion, making sure you get into pits.

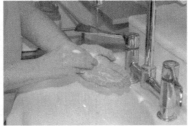

8. Rub the tip of fingers against palm of hands in a circular motion (to clean nails).

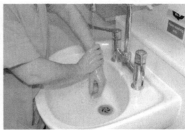

9. Wash the wrists.

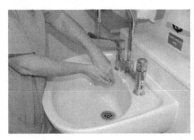

10. Rinse hands thoroughly.

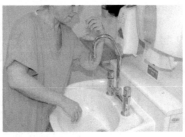

11. Turn off taps with elbows.

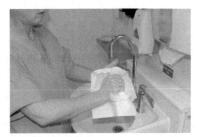

12. Dry hands with a single use towel.

4. <u>Hospital Wards, the Day Unit and Intensive Care</u>

The in-patient ward, its staff and routines

Only a small proportion of oral and maxillofacial patients will need hospital admission and an overnight stay in a ward. These will mostly be receiving major surgery for cancer, facial trauma, or orthognathics.

Each ward has a sister or charge nurse in overall control with any number of registered nurses, often known as 'staff nurses'. Assisting the nurses will be several health care assistants who help with a variety of tasks, such as assisting patients wash, bedmaking, and distribution of meals. There will also be domestic 'housekeeping' staff who will be involved with cleaning, laundry and taking charge of the ward kitchen and ordering of meals from the main hospital kitchen.

Each patient admitted should have a named nurse who will be in charge of their nursing care on any particular shift. A patient's named nurse should know about the patient's condition in some detail and be able to give a personalised nursing service. Obviously, one nurse cannot be on duty for 24 hours so that when there is a change in shift there is 'a changeover' where the nurse hands over the care of the patient to the new nurse, usually referring to their written nursing records.

The patient turn over on acute surgical wards is often high and together with staffing problems, it is common for the named nurse to change frequently. It is therefore essential that the patients are visited often by the medical staff and the nurse should be involved in any discussion about patient care and kept up to date with plans for their management.

Somewhere by each bed should be written the name of the consultant or specialty who has overall responsibility for that patient. There will be a note trolley on the ward containing the patient's medical notes, which are the responsibility of the medical staff; an entry should be made each time a patient is visited by the medical staff or management changed. There will also be a folder containing the nursing notes and, usually in a separate trolley, the drugs chart of each patient.

The nurse should be cognisant of all the patient's problems, treatment, concerns and expectations. She or he will also take particular note of the social background and details of home support after the patient has been discharged from the ward. There will be a nursing 'care plan' which will be written in the nursing notes. We find that for writing reports and

Indications for Ward admission in OMFS
1. Major surgery requiring specialized post op surgical care
2. Multiple injuries
3. Mandibular fractures awaiting urgent theatre
4. Mid face fractures for post-operative care or observation
5. Head injuries for observation where there has been loss of consciousness or nausea
6. Routine Surgery under GA with a co-existing medical problem such as poorly controlled diabetes, cardiac disease or bleeding diathesis
7. Routine surgery which cannot be done as day stay because patient:-
a. lives a long distance away
b. will not be accompanied home
c. will be alone for the first 24 hours post surgery
d. has body mass index + 35

statements, sometime after the event, it is often the nursing notes which are the most complete, legible and useful.

On admission, each patient will have an identity band placed around a wrist. This will have their name, date of birth and NHS/hospital number printed on it. There will also be a bar code. The identity band should be checked each time medication is given, blood or other samples taken, or any procedure undertaken. The patient is also asked to confirm their name and date of birth verbally, and the bar code is scanned when observations are taken. All this is to protect against identity errors.

The nurses will also record the patient's 'observations' (known as 'obs'). These comprise their 'vital signs': blood pressure, pulse rate, temperature, respiratory rate, level of consciousness, pain score (from 0 to 3), and oxygen saturation. These used to be recorded on a chart at the end of each patient's bed but are now more likely to be recorded on a mobile phone and transmitted to a computer, which will work out the patient's MEWS (modified early warning score). See Post-Operative Care chapter for the significance of MEWS score.

In addition, there may be other specific observations, which may be requested in certain circumstances. In particular, a fluid balance chart will record the oral and parenteral intake of fluid and urine output; neurological observations will be made for patients who have received head injuries, or eye observations for patients who have received surgery for peri-orbital fractures.

Nursing shifts usually change at about 8.00am, 2pm and 10 pm and you should ensure that you visit the ward at least once during every nursing shift. It is not uncommon for nurses to work 12-hour shifts; this appears to be popular as it gives them 3 clear days off each week. It is not uncommon for nurses to work excessive hours. Often they will make themselves available for the 'nursing bank' where they will work extra shifts above their contracted hours to fill in for shortages.

The medical staff should have a formal ward round of the patients in the morning with the consultants or the specialist registrar and a visit to the patients at the end of the working day (after 5.00 p.m.). When on call, make a short visit after the night shift has come on at about 10 pm. With the occasional patient who is in hospital for a prolonged stay and in whom there is little change in their condition, the last two visits will be very short. For post-operative cases, particularly major ones, it will be more prolonged and the senior staff will probably visit the patient twice or more per day with you. In either case, ensure that you are there to receive and understand their instructions for management.

It is important that sufficient information is passed onto colleagues for the patients to be looked after adequately when you are off duty. 'Handover' is best carried out at the patient's bedside, but this may not always be practical. Information given verbally can be supplemented by a written note. It is useful to pass on a written management plan at weekends.

Prior to operation, the patient may be admitted on the morning of surgery to a 'surgical admission lounge' from where they will go to the operating theatre. Consent for operation should have been done beforehand, but the surgeon should see the patient before theatre again, as should the anaesthetist. A nurse will check that the patient has given consent and that they are appropriately starved. They will accompany them to the operating theatre.

When the patient is fit to be discharged from the hospital, the named nurse will arrange for the outpatient appointment to be made. They will communicate with the district nurse should any nursing be required at home; for example, change of dressings. They will also communicate with relatives to arrange collection of the patient from the ward.

Besides the trained nurses and healthcare support workers, there are many other professionals, based on, or visiting the wards, who participate in the patient's care. The ward clerk will make sure that the records are present for the admission if the hospital does not yet use electronic records. Once a day the ward pharmacist will visit; he or she will check the drug chart and make sure that the prescribed drugs are available. Pharmacists are a valuable additional safeguard against prescribing errors; if there are any doubts or queries, they will write them on the charts. Doubts by the pharmacist or nurse about drugs or their dosage should always be considered very seriously.

Each morning, a phlebotomist will visit the ward to take blood for routine tests, etc. In order for them to help you, it will therefore be necessary to make sure requests have been made through the clinical records system the night before. In some areas such as Accident and Emergency, Acute Surgical Assessment Unit, High Dependency and Intensive Care, the nurses will have been trained to place intravenous lines and take blood samples. A physiotherapist will visit each ward; they usually visit patients on the request of the named nurse. It is unlikely in OMFS that patients will have locomotor problems and need help with mobilisation, but post-operative patients, particularly those who have had pre-existing chest disease or are smokers, will be given chest physiotherapy on request.

The dietician will visit the ward to give advice and prescribe nutritional supplements to patients who are having difficulties with eating. In our specialty, there may be the occasional patient who has inter-maxillary fixation or, more likely, patients having enteral tube feeding if they are 'nil by mouth' following oral reconstruction consequent on ablative cancer surgery.

For most patients on a surgical ward, the day will start early. This may be as early as 6.00 am with the arrival of a nurse on the night shift who will do the early morning drug round or administering intra-venous medication. They will want these time-consuming tasks finished before the day staff arrives at 7.00 am and they will need to spend half an hour handing over the patients before they go off duty at 7.30 and before the doctors arrive to see their patients. In addition, the nurses will need to do their first round of observations and all intra-venous cannulae will need to be flushed with saline to ensure they are still patent with no surrounding erythema. Intra-venous fluid bags may need changing and for patients with urinary catheters, these will need checking; urine bags will need changing and output measured and recorded.

Soon after 7.00 am, the domestic staff become apparent. They will start by taking away all the patient's bedside water jugs and beakers and replacing them with fresh. They will go round delivering the daily menu cards and filling them in for those who need help and then serve breakfast from the ward kitchen, which is likely to be limited to cereal, fruit and toast with coffee or tea. The main meal of the day will be at lunchtime and this and the evening meal will come from the central hospital kitchen and will be served by the domestic staff, assisted by the health care assistants and sometimes by the nurses.

After breakfast, the domestics will start cleaning and the health care assistants will change all the bedclothes of anybody who gets out of the bed. When any patient leaves, the whole area around their bed will be mopped, and all surfaces cleaned with alcohol wipes, and bed and mattress covers cleaned. Mid-morning and afternoon the domestics will do a coffee and tea round.

Visiting will normally be in the afternoon from 2.00 to 9.00 p.m. but no-one visiting outside this time will be turned away and on Saturday and Sunday afternoon visitors will arrive from far and wide and there will be loud and lively conversation.

Most of those admitted for oral or maxillofacial surgery will be patients receiving ablative cancer operations, who need specialised post-operative care, trauma patients, those receiving orthognathic surgery or those who have severe oro-facial sepsis. Some patients may be admitted because they have co-existing medical problems and are having a general anaesthetic; for example, poorly controlled diabetics, or patients with cardiac disease or bleeding diathesis. Sometimes there may be social reasons, such as having no one to take them home after surgery or they live a long way from the hospital. Some patients may be admitted because they are too obese for a general anaesthetic as a day stay (body mass index +35).

Most patients will be fit to go home when they can eat, drink, pass urine, their pain has been controlled, and they can get home and look after themselves or have someone else to help. If they do not and they are infirm, the social workers may need to be involved and an occupational therapy assessment may be needed to find out what level of support they need. This should ideally be predicted in advance, in order to avoid unnecessary delay, and the bed being 'blocked' by a patient who does not need acute surgical care anymore.

Before a patient is discharged home, ensure that the patient has an outpatient review appointment (but only if necessary), that appropriate medication has been prescribed (particularly analgesics if they have had surgery), and post-operative instructions given. The patient's GP should be informed of the discharge by completing the electronic discharge document on a hospital computer.

The Day Surgery Unit

Most oral and maxillofacial surgery, particularly dento-alveolar, can be carried out with local anaesthetic, usually in an outpatient facility, sometimes with sedation. On those occasions where a general anaesthetic is prescribed, it will usually be done in the day unit.

The unit will usually have facilities for patients to be seated prior to surgery and who will normally be recovered afterwards on the same trolley they were on during the operation. Patients will normally walk in to the anaesthetic room. The whole flow of patients is organised to maximise efficiency and turnover.

The most important consideration is choosing which patients and cases are suitable. All patients having surgery under anaesthetic will be seen by a nurse at a pre-operative assessment clinic. They will follow a pro-forma which will include all aspects of their medical and social history and will decide whether they are suitable for a day admission or they need to be admitted overnight to an in-patient ward. The American Society of Anaesthetists in 1962 devised the Physical Status Classification System range from a Grade 1 (fit and healthy) to Grade 6 (dead). For day surgery, the patient must be ASA grade 1 or 2, although most of our day patients will be ASA grade 1.

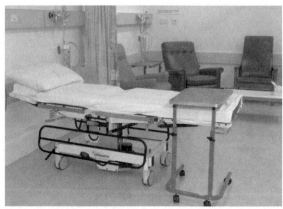

Most patients wait in chairs and transfer to a trolley before surgery; they stay on the same trolley for surgery and recovery

Patients who are grossly obese may have an airway problem after a general anaesthetic and so must be carefully monitored post-operatively. It is therefore usually considered unsafe to do day surgery under anaesthetic for patients whose body mass index is above 35. However, some hospitals have removed this requirement.

The success of day surgery depends on good post-operative analgesia. In practical terms, this involves infiltration of long-acting local anaesthetic, bupivacaine 0.5% with 1:200,000 adrenaline next to the operation site; this will give 6 to 8 hours of analgesia. Diclofenac may be given before, during, or after surgery; the slow release formulation should give 12 hours of comfort. This is usually followed up by ibuprofen 400 mg. t.d.s. orally with the advice to the patient that this is taken regularly for the first three days, as pain is better anticipated with analgesia rather than reacted to.

The Intensive Care Unit

The Intensive Care Unit (ICU) provides a higher level of monitoring and support for seriously ill or deteriorating patients than is available on the general wards. This will include mechanical ventilation and complex support for patients with multiple organ failure. Most patients on ICU have cardiovascular or respiratory problems, electrolyte and renal malfunction, or depressed consciousness. In many cases, this may have been triggered or exacerbated by sepsis of one sort or another.

ICU may also provide an outreach service to advise about patients on the wards who have a physiological abnormality which is at risk of deteriorating. The intention is to help reverse this and avoid an Intensive Care admission. Patients may be referred directly to the ICU outreach service by ward nurses. This will be triggered by a scoring system based on a chart called the Modified Early Warning System, which has been shown to be an accurate predictor of clinical deterioration (see Post-Operative Care chapter). Patients receive intensive care only if they are likely to benefit from it, not just because they are seriously ill. They will not benefit from it if death from their presenting condition is inevitable, for example uncontrolled cancer or end-stage cardiac failure.

Admission to ICU may be from the Accident and Emergency Department, from the general wards, or from the operating theatre. Some patients may be booked into ICU in advance if they are having major surgery and they have serious co-morbidity such as cardiac or respiratory disease.

On 'the unit', patients are looked after by the specialist 'intensivists' who are usually specialist anaesthetists. They are assisted by a large team of other professionals, most numerous of whom are the specialist ICU nurses. Each patient will have a nurse solely assigned to them. Where surgeons are involved with the patients, there will be shared care; the surgical team should visit each day to contribute advice from the surgical perspective. All treatment orders and prescriptions requested by the surgeons should be formally written by the intensivists; this avoids any confusion.

Patients who require oral and maxillofacial surgery care shared with intensive care usually fall mostly within two categories. First, patients who are receiving major resections of cancers of the head and neck, often with soft tissue flap repair, and second, patients with multiple injuries which include face and jaw injury. Occasionally, we may have a patient in the ICU who has major oro-facial sepsis, usually caused by a dental abscess.

Most patients having major head and neck cancer resection will be transferred from the recovery unit in theatres directly to the ward for post-operative care. However, they may go to ICU if they have co-existing severe cardiac or respiratory disease, especially where post-operative ventilation is desirable. Similarly, most patients with facial injuries will not need intensive care as facial injuries are not life threatening unless there is severe bleeding or airways obstruction. However, patients with multiple injuries, particularly of the head or chest, may need intensive care. The facial injuries are usually dealt with when the life-threatening injuries have been stabilised; the maxillofacial team will have to liaise with the intensivists over the best time to operate.

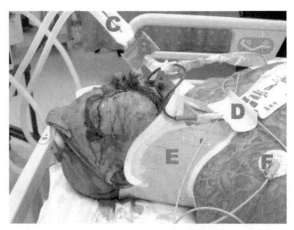

A patient admitted to ICU 3 hours after a motorcycle accident. His only injuries were a fractured arm and maxilla. He has been heavily sedated with Propofol and is being artificially ventilated through an oral endotracheal tube because of massive facial swelling which would otherwise obstruct his airway. A. endotracheal tube B. air filter C. breathing circuit to ventilator D. bag attached to gastric tube to aspirate stomach contents to prevent regurgitation E. rigid neck collar to stabilize cervical spine (all patients with severe facial injuries are assumed to have cervical spine injuries until they have been X rayed or CT scanned and cleared by an orthopaedic surgeon) F. ECG electrode. I operated on him a week later & he was discharged home 2 days after that.

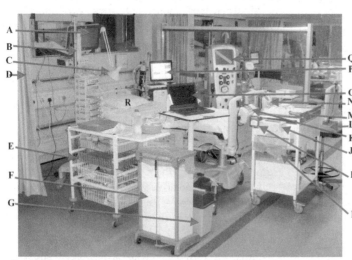

A. Video monitor for ECG., blood pressure, PO_2, CO_2, temperature, venous pressure, airways gases and pressure
B. Drip stand for infusions
C. Lamp

D. Curtain for visual privacy
E. Equipment and materials trolley
F. Clinical waste bag
G. Sharps disposal bin
H. Personal protective disposable aprons
I. Alcohol hand rub
J. Disposable examination gloves
K. Mattress pump controller (prevent pressure sores)
L. Stool for nurse
M. Calculator and observation charts
N. Flowtron controller (controls calf compression to decrease deep vein thrombosis risk)
O. Computer to access patient records (blood and imaging results and reports)
P. Ventilator
Q. Dialysis machine
R. Bed

Empty bed on ICU awaiting patient

5. <u>Preparation for Operation and Consent</u>

Procedures before planned surgery

Preparation for planned surgery will start in the outpatient clinic with the discussion between surgeon and patient about the indications, contraindications, and alternatives to surgery. Questions will be answered and consent will be obtained.

Once the patient has a date for surgery, if they are to be admitted to a ward or day unit for surgery with a general anaesthetic, they will be seen by a registered nurse who will carry out the process often called 'pre-clerking' or 'care planning'. This ensures that the patient is fully prepared, that the appropriate investigations are carried out and that they know what to expect and where to come and when. If day surgery is planned, the nurse will check that their physical health and social circumstances concord with the accepted criteria for day surgery.

This will involve going through, with the patient, a fairly complicated care plan document, which includes a detailed assessment of their current and previous medical and social history, a systems review of symptoms they may have which might indicate any underlying cardiac or respiratory disease, and a social history which might have a bearing on their discharge from hospital and post-operative care. The assessment will usually include routine observations such as blood pressure, pulse, height, weight and body mass index. Current medication will be listed. The patient will be given instructions about not eating and drinking prior to surgery; the length of time they should be starved will depend upon the surgery and local policy.

Investigations will be ordered by the nurse under a protocol which will almost certainly follow the guidelines of the National Institute for Health & Care Excellence (NICE). This should ensure that no one should present on the day of surgery without the essential investigations having been done and checked, and resources should not have been wasted on requesting unnecessary tests. There is no point in carrying out a special test at some inconvenience and expense if it is unlikely to change the management of the patient.

On the day of surgery, there will be further checks made by the admitting nurse. It will need to be confirmed when they last ate or drank; they will need to be fitted with an identity band, and the consent form will be returned and signed. The patient will be dressed

Investigation	*Indication*
ECG	Pre-existing cardiac or respiratory disease
	Smoker over 40
	Anyone over 60
Chest X Ray	Is almost never needed but may be requested if there is existing cardiac or respiratory disease
Full blood count	Over 60
	Anyone for major surgery with significant blood loss
	More minor surgery with some blood loss with history of cardiac disease
Urea & electrolytes	Renal disease
	Diabetics
	Taking diuretics
Serum glucose	Diabetics
	On steroids
	Severe sepsis
Coagulation screen	Anti coagulants (INR)
	Liver disease
	Family or past history of problem bleeding
Sickle/ Hb. electrophoresis	Ethnic groups at risk if not previously tested or no history of previous anaesthetic if counselled and consented. North African, West African, South/sub Saharan African, Afro Caribbean, Eastern Mediterranean, Middle Eastern, Asian.

Pre-operative investigations in OMFS

Thank you for asking me to see Mr   concerning the swelling in his
lower lip.

Clinically this looks like a mucous extravasation cyst due to trauma from his
teeth. I have advised him that this will continue to recur if it is not removed so
we are making arrangements to carry this out under local anaesthetic. I have
advised Mr   that his lip will be swollen, sore and uncomfortable for
about a week afterwards and there is a small risk of some numbness of the
vermilion of the lower lip due to the proximity of the small nerves which supply
sensation to it.

Yours sincerely

It is helpful to mention them in the letter to the GP and send a copy to the patient

in a theatre gown, decorative finger rings will be taped, and dentures or spectacles removed and kept in a safe place, usually the bedside locker. Patients will be seen by the anaesthetist for a pre-operative assessment and by someone from the surgical team who will need to find out if there are any further questions or explanations which should be attended to; this will be confirmed on the consent form. If the operation is outside the mouth, the operation site should be marked with a skin marking pen and the admission document signed to confirm that this has been done. You should ensure that you visit the ward or day unit with the surgeon in charge and familiarise yourself with their case history and examine them if you have not already had the opportunity to do so.

Consent for hospital treatment

It is sometimes not well understood that consent for treatment is much more than placing the signature on a form. It should involve the patient being informed of what treatment can be provided, what the alternatives are, what the risks are, and the side-effects as well as the benefits. There should include a discussion about the consequences of no treatment. The patient must be capable of absorbing the information and making choices offered to them. The consent form is a useful adjunct to this process but is not the be all and end all as some might consider it to be. Comprehensive notes, written at the time, provide evidence that a robust consenting process has been used.

The standards which are used in an acute NHS trust for obtaining consent are important to the National Health Service Litigation Authority (NHSLA) which provides indemnity to NHS trusts under their Clinical Negligence Scheme for Trusts (CNST) scheme. The gold standard is that the patient's consent is obtained by the clinician who is going to perform the procedure. However, failing this, consent can be obtained from somebody who has been trained to do it and can discuss the benefits, risks and side-effects of the procedure and its alternatives.

The Consent Forms

Form 1: Patient agreement to investigation or treatment

Form 2: For parental agreement investigation or treatment for a child or young person

Form 3: Patient/ parental agreement for investigation or treatment which does not require a general anaesthetic. (procedures where consciousness is not impaired)

Form 4: Form for adults who are unable to consent to investigation or treatment

---

Some Principles of Consent

The decision must be the patient's.

Patient must have the capacity to make a decision; it must be assumed that a patient does have the capacity unless it is established that he does not.

The patient should be warned of any material risks of proposed treatment and of alternatives.

The doctor should be aware which particular risks the patient would regard as material.

Children under 16 may have the capacity to consent to treatment.

A parent can consent to treatment for a child.

A person aged 16 can be presumed to have capacity to consent.

No one can give consent on behalf of another adult.

Patient should be told of the diagnosis, proposed treatment, its risks & complications, alternative treatments, their risks and complications and the consequence of no treatment.

Patient must give consent voluntarily.

The surgeon should be aware if that patient will be likely to attach significance to any particular risk. We believe, therefore, that getting consent for surgery is not a suitable job to be delegated to a new trainee.

The forms used to confirm that consent has been given are fairly standard in acute NHS trusts; they are very far from perfect. It is unfair to ask a patient to sign straight away in the clinic as there is too much on the form for them to read and it gives them insufficient time to digest the discussion that has taken place. Most patients, in our experience, do not bother to read the forms (often they don't have their spectacles with them). We prefer to fill in our part of a form and ask the patient to take it away to sign later and bring it back. However, about a third of patients forget to bring it back with them and we have often to fill out another.

Initially, you will be too inexperienced to consent patients for operation other than for very minor procedures such as a biopsy. The consent form itself should be written in terms that the patient can understand, so abbreviations and dental charting should not be used. The forms themselves have a top copy of the information recorded by the clinician, which tears off for the patient to keep a record of their own.

The consent form 4 is used for adult patients who are unable to consent for treatment. This is slightly more complicated and those who treat such patients should know the law and, in particular, the Mental Incapacity Act. Usually the consultant will deal with all such cases in OMFS and these are very few. In our practice, they are most frequently severe trauma cases where the patient is sedated and intubated when we arrive. Usually our job is first aid in the shape of a tracheostomy, arrest of haemorrhage, suturing of lacerations, the removal of loose teeth and stabilisation of facial fractures. In these circumstances, only the urgent treatment should be carried out and it must be in the patient's best interest. In some hospitals, the OMF surgeons provide a tracheostomy service for patients who are already intubated and ventilated and therefore unable to give consent; consent form 4 will be used in all these cases.

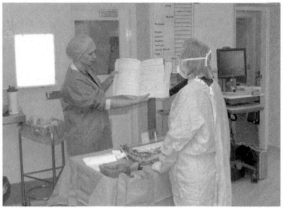

Nurses in theatre check the consent form to ensure the patient is getting the right operation.

Procedure	Intended benefit	Serious or frequently occurring risk	Our comment
Surgical removal of impacted third molar tooth	To prevent further pain or infection	Numbness or tingling of lip or tongue, <u>probably</u> temporary	Risk of permanent numbness about 2% tongue 0.25% lip
Incisional biopsy of swelling in mouth	For diagnosis of swelling		No need to mention swelling, discomfort or bleeding on the form. The patient should be verbally warned of these but they are not risks; rather they are side effects to be expected and are not serious
Excisional biopsy of swelling	To remove the lump and for diagnosis		
Suture of laceration of face	To close wound to achieve best appearance	None (leave blank)	
Open reduction & fixation of fracture of zygoma (malar)	Restore contour of face, improve jaw movement, improve chance of recovery of face numbness, improve double vision	Bleed into eye socket	Very rare but should be mentioned as this can threaten vision

Consent issues for some common operations

6. <u>The Operating Theatre</u>

Operating theatre procedure and ritual

The operating theatre suite will have many individual theatres. Usually, these will be dedicated to specific disciplines or groups. Orthopaedics usually has its own dedicated theatres with laminar air ventilation in which bacteria free filtered air is circulated under pressure into the operating site so that contaminated air is removed away from the patient. This may reduce the incidence of airborne infection, which can be disastrous in joint replacement surgery.

Each theatre will have its own anaesthetic room where the patient is prepared and anaesthetised; a preparation ('prep') room where the instruments and other equipment are prepared and laid out on trolleys; a 'scrub' room where surgeons, assistants, and nurses wash their hands and put on gowns and gloves. There will be a 'dirty' area where instruments and drapes are taken after the operation and where pathology specimens from cancer surgery are taken to be orientated and pinned to a corkboard for the pathologist. Somewhere in the suite there will also be store rooms, staff rest rooms, a kitchen, offices, a reception area and recovery rooms where the patients are taken immediately after surgery. All the theatres will be air-conditioned with about 20 changes of air per hour so that airborne bacteria shed from the staff or patients' skin or even from a dirty wound will be swiftly carried out.

A few days before each operating session, a list of patients will have been prepared, usually by the consultant's secretary or booked admissions team. The patients will be listed in order of booking time with

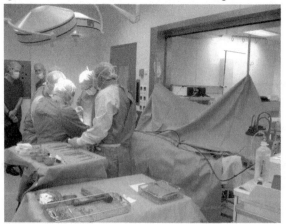

Theatre. The surgeon, assistant and scrub nurse wear sterile gowns; there is an unsterile 'runner' who fetches additional equipment.

their ages, hospital number and procedure recorded; there may be additional special theatre requirements added.

Each theatre in the suite will have a nurse in charge who may be a staff nurse, sister or charge nurse. When the anaesthetist and nurses are ready and the surgeon has arrived, the nurse in charge will inform the theatre receptionist to send for the patient, who will be escorted from the ward by a porter and a ward nurse. On arrival, the patient will be booked in at the theatre reception, their identity will be checked, both verbally and by looking at their wrist band, and the consent form will be checked. They will then be taken to the anaesthetic room. It is here that all the first part of the World Health Organization (WHO) checklist, which has three stages, will be carried out. The first, known as 'sign in', takes place before the anaesthetic is induced. Once 'sign in' has occurred, the anaesthetic can begin.

The anaesthetic room contains all the equipment necessary to put the patient to sleep. The anaesthetist will be assisted by an Operating Department Practitioner (ODP) or an anaesthetic nurse. While the patient is being anaesthetised, the surgical instruments are prepared in the 'prep' room by a nurse who has 'scrubbed'. This 'scrub nurse' will prepare the sterile instruments while an unsterile nurse, the 'runner', will hand things to her, touching only the unsterile part of the wrappings. The instruments used in any operation by a particular surgeon will be kept on a list in a card index in the theatre or computer, so the nurse will know which instruments to prepare.

The ODP or anaesthetic nurse will draw up the drugs, unwrap and pass equipment, and set up the monitoring equipment. When anaesthetised, the patient can be transferred to the operating theatre, and the operation begins. In the theatre itself, the second stage of the WHO checklist, known as 'time out', takes place.

The surgeon and assistant should scrub while the patient is in the anaesthetic room, so they are ready to start as soon as the patient is on the table. During the operation, the ODP or anaesthetic nurse will assist the anaesthetist while the scrub nurse passes instruments to the surgeon. The runner should remain in theatre and fetch equipment and instruments as required. You should scrub and take part in the surgery in whatever manner instructed by the surgeon.

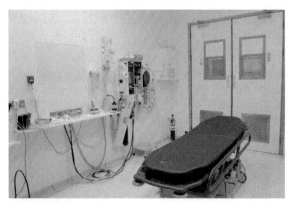

Anaesthetic room

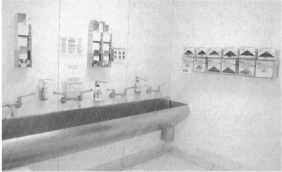

The scrub room. It is equipped with elbow operated taps. There are dispensers on the wall containing disposable nail brushes and sponges impregnated with chlorhexidine, PCMX or iodine and separate dispensers. Sterile gloves are on the wall.

After the operation, the final stage of the WHO checklist, known as 'sign out', is made. The senior surgeon will probably wish to write up the operating notes himself. For day cases, a TTA (to take away) prescription should be made, usually on the computer, with an electronic discharge for the GP, usually completed by the trainee.

There are several operating theatre rituals and conventions you will need to know about and adhere to; these are principally designed to reduce cross infection. The evidence for their efficacy is variable, so you find that there will be some slight variation between hospitals. You may find that some hospitals still require patients to remove all items of their own clothing, cover their hair, and take off any jewellery. It is usual practice to tape rings to prevent them being dislodged and lost.

You will enter the theatre suite through a door directly into a changing room where you should change into cotton 'scrubs'; these will be freshly laundered but socially clean rather than sterile.

WHO Surgical Safety Checklist - Part 1 Sign in

Patient has confirmed:-

Identity, site, procedure, consent

Site marked/not applicable

Anaesthesia safety check completed

Pulse oximeter on patient and functioning

Does patient have:-

Known allergy: yes or no

Difficult airway/aspiration risk

No

Yes and equipment/assistance available

Risk of >500ml blood loss

No

Yes and adequate IV access and fluids

WHO Surgical Safety Checklist - Part 2 Time out

All team members introduce themselves by name and role

Surgeon, anaesthetist & nurse verbally confirm:-

Patient, Site, Procedure

Anticipated critical events:-

Surgeon reviews: Critical or unexpected steps, operative duration, anticipated blood loss

Anaesthesia review: any specific patient concerns
Nursing reviews: sterility confirmed, any equipment issues or other concerns

Has antibiotic prophylaxis been given in last 60 minutes? Yes/not applicable

Is essential imaging displayed? Yes/not applicable

WHO Surgical Safety Checklist - Part 3 Sign out

Name of procedure recorded

Instrument, sponge & needle counts correct or not applicable

How the specimen is labeled

Whether there are any equipment problems to be addressed

Surgeon, anaesthetist & nurse review key concerns for recovery & management

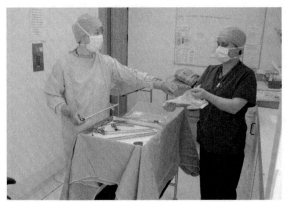

The sterile scrub nurse is preparing the instruments in the 'prep' room. The unsterile 'runner' is passing equipment by holding the unsterile outer wrapping.

Scrubbing and gowning

Staff who wear jewellery should remove it in theatre, but a single wedding ring is usually not removed. A ring worn beneath a glove does not contribute to cross infection, although it may lead to an increase in glove perforation. False finger nails, however, do harbour pathogenic bacteria and should not be worn.

The process of pre-operative hand washing and donning surgical gloves and sterile gown is known as 'scrubbing up'. Finger nails should be kept short, and the first wash of the day should include a thorough clean of the finger nails using a stick or brush. Thereafter, the hands should be washed using chlorhexidine gluconate 4%, 7.5% povidone iodine scrub solution or PCMX (Parachlorometaxylenol), using the technique previously described for two minutes. The supplied nail brushes should not be used on the skin as they can cause abrasions. Theatre gowns and drapes are now mostly disposable, as these are less permeable to epithelial cells and bacteria shed from staff or patients than the formerly used linen. Once you have scrubbed, you should not touch any non-sterile surface or object. If you accidentally touch something with your hand, it is easier to put on a second glove than to change.

Below is demonstrated the sequence of 'scrubbing' for surgery. It involves placing a sterile gown and gloves, opened, on the trolley, washing hands, putting on the gown followed by the gloves and getting someone to tie up the gown behind. Once scrubbed, you must touch nothing unsterile with your hands or body.

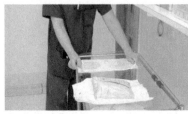

1. Tear open a gown pack touching only the outer wrap.

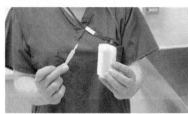

2. Open the glove packet touching only the outer wrap.

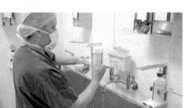

4. Clean beneath nails and scrub them but only for the first wash of the day. Do not brush other skin.

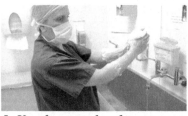

5. Use the same hand movements as on 'hand cleaning' section but go up towards elbows.

3. Antiseptic scrub solutions are impregnated into a sponge with a scrubbing brush & a nail cleaning tool.

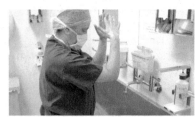

6. Turn off tap with elbows and let water drain off arms.

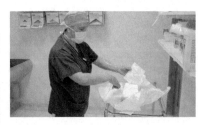

7. Open the gown pack; touch the outside of the inner wrap only. Take a paper towel.

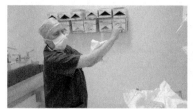

8. Dry the hands first moving up to elbows.

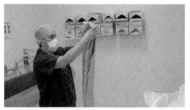

9. Take the gown, hold at the top and allow it to unroll; touch only the inside.

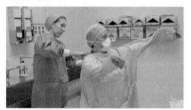

10. Push arms into gown. Runner pulls gown up arms from inside and ties gown behind.

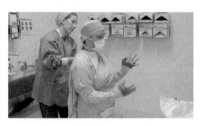

11. Hands protrude out of gown. We are going to use an 'open' technique to don gloves.

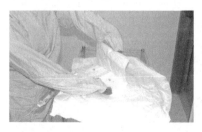

12. The glove packet being opened. They are packed with the cuff folded back.

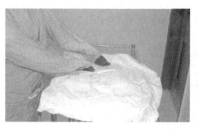

13. The cuff of the left glove is picked up, touching through the gown.

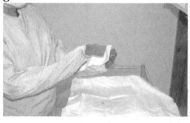

14. Fold the left glove over the left hand , pulling with the right hand touching the inside of the cuff area.

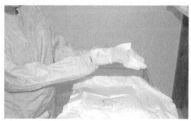

15. Pull the glove on.

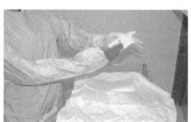

16. Pick up the second glove.

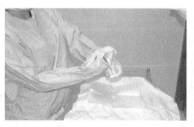

17. Pull on the right glove; you can touch this anywhere with the gloved left hand.

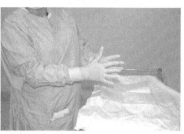

18. Complete.

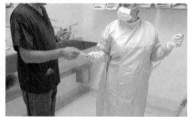

19. Now tie the waistband. Hand the card attached to the waistband to someone who is not scrubbed.

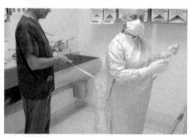

20. Twirl around so that the band goes around your waist and the back of the gown is closed.

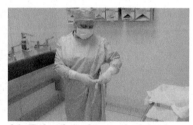

21. Take the other end of the band and tie it.

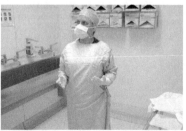

22. Ready for theatre.

7. **Post-Operative Patient Care**

The routine post-operative care process

Following surgery, the patient will be transferred from the operating theatre to the recovery area of theatres when they are sufficiently awake. The anaesthetist will hand over the patient to the recovery staff and keep overall responsibility for the patient until they leave the theatre suite. A recovery nurse will monitor the patient's welfare, particularly their airway, and when satisfied the patients are well enough will ask the anaesthetist for permission for them to return to the ward or day unit. They will then call for a ward nurse and porter to take the patient. The recovery nurse will hand over to the ward nurse.

The surgical team, which includes you, should hand over any specific instructions or warnings concerning the surgery that the recovery nurse should know about.

After the operating session has finished, you should visit the patient on the ward to check for any problems and contact the patient's named nurse to ensure they know of any special issues regarding their care. In most routine cases, this contact will only need to be brief, but frequently patients may be admitted to non-specialist wards where the nurses are not experienced in looking after OMFS patients and you will need to explain the surgery to them. The anaesthetist will also visit the patient on the ward. This is usually a brief attendance to ensure that there is no problem with the airway and that the analgesia they have prescribed is sufficient.

Post-operative pain management is very important. Pain is much better anticipated than reacted to. It is important for you to check that this has been given and that the patients are comfortable.

The patient should be visited at the end of the working day to check on them again and in the late evening after the night nursing staff have come on to ensure that they are familiar with the case. The surgical team should ensure that the nurse knows what surgery has been done, any complications that might arise, and the plan for recovery. This is most important if the patient is an 'outlier' from your usual ward and the nurses are not familiar with OMFS.

The nurses should undertake routine observations (known as obs). These used to be recorded on paper charts (and may be still in some hospitals) but are

Routine patient observations
Level of consciousness
Respiratory rate
Temperature
Pulse rate
Blood pressure
Oxygen saturation
Pain score

usually done on a computer which can be accessed on a screen in the ward. The computer will work out their Medical Early Warning (MEWS) score. This gives a prediction of if a patient is becoming medically unwell and at risk of deterioration. More of this later. The surgical team should look at the patient's 'obs' when they visit them on the ward. Wounds should be inspected for bleeding or excessive swelling; an enquiry should be made about pain (which is not acceptable) or discomfort (which is to be expected). The patient should be encouraged to sit up or sit out of bed and walk as soon as possible, as early ambulation is desirable to prevent atelectasis (peripheral lung collapse) and venous thrombosis.

Each morning, the surgical team should visit each patient on a ward round. You will go round with the consultant or specialist registrar; this visit should include the patient's named nurse who will report on their progress. Pain, fluid intake (and output if it is a major case), eating, pain control should all be checked. The observations record should be checked. Intravenous lines should be checked to ensure they are patent and if there is any sign of inflammation. If the patient is taking an adequate oral intake, they may be removed. Any surgical drains that have been placed should be checked to ensure they are working, i.e. that they are not blocked or have lost their vacuum. If they are working, but there has been little drainage, they may be removed.

If the patient has pain adequately controlled, has passed urine, is eating and drinking and has a responsible adult to accompany them, then they can probably be discharged home. Follow up care should be discussed and arranged; complications and side effects should be discussed. Any medication to take home should be prescribed and a discharge pro-forma completed for the patient's General Medical

Observation	Units	21 Sep 2018 05:55	20 Sep 2018 21:02	20 Sep 2018 10:24	20 Sep 2018 06:24	19 Sep 2018 21:28	19 Sep 2018 17:12	19 Sep 2018 11:31
Site	-	Lincoln	Lincoln	Lincoln	Lincoln	Lincoln	Lincoln	Lincoln
Location	-	Surgical Admissions Lounge	Surgical Admissions Lounge	Surgical Admissions Lounge	Surgical Admissions Lounge	Surgical Admissions Lounge	Surgical Admissions Lounge	Surgical Admissions Lounge
Bed	-	Bay 4 Bed 15	Bay 4 Bed 15	Bay 4 Bed 15	Bay 4 Bed 15	Bay 4 Bed 15	Bay 4 Bed 15	Bay 4 Bed 15
Pulse	BPM	79	75	75	79	70	72	72
Respiration	br/min	16	16	12	16	16	12	16
Temperature	Celsius	37.2	36.9	36.8	37.5	37.3	36.7	36.9
Systolic BP	mmHg	142	133	122	124	128	121	124
Diastolic BP	mmHg	83	76	72	71	81	72	73
O2 Saturation	%	96	96	96	95	96	95	94
O2 Supplement	L/min	0	0	0	0	0	0	0
CNS Response	-	Alert	Alert	Alert	Alert	Alert	Alert	Alert
Pain Score	Score	1	0	0	0	0	0	0
Hypercapnia (Scale 2)	-	No	No	No	No	No	No	No
NEWS Score	-	0	0	0	1	0	1	1
Observer	-							

Patient's 'obs' displayed on a screen in the ward. The computer has worked out the MEWS score. With a score now of 0 the main screen will inform the nurses that this patient will only need observations done 12 hourly.

Checks before a patient can be discharged

Patient can eat & drink

Has passed urine

Apyrexial

Adequate pain control with oral analgesics

Is self-caring or has adequate help

Has transport home or can be accompanied

Practitioner. You will have to do this, most probably on-line, usually with the patient being given a paper copy. This should include details of the problem, diagnosis, findings, follow up and medication.

Throughout the process, you should record progress in the patient's notes, including when they have been visited, by whom, changes in condition or management and the surgical plan.

Your role in dealing with complications

A complication is an adverse event which may increase the morbidity of a patient following any treatment, most commonly, but not necessarily, a surgical operation. We seek to minimise the risk of complications through good pre-operative planning, sound surgery, and meticulous post-operative care. You will be part of this.

Complications may be classified as local or systemic and as immediate, delayed or late. We will discuss delayed or late systemic complications. Immediate complications will occur in the operating theatre where there will be a senior surgeon present to deal with them. Local complications (i.e. at the operation site) will be part of your learning within the job. The next paragraph is the most important in this chapter.

We will thus discuss medical complications of surgery that OMFS patients are likely to sustain. The reason for discussing these is to allow you to understand what may go wrong and the principle of dealing with them. You will be part of the surgical team and will assist in post-operative management, but at no stage must you, as a dentist, initiate the treatment of medical complications or manage them without the full intervention of the responsible consultant or medically qualified registrar. If you see a patient with a complication, you must tell your consultant or specialist registrar.

The patients most at risk of developing systemic complications are the elderly and medically unfit, such as those who have pre-existing cardiovascular or respiratory disease or are immunocompromised, such as diabetics. The risks are increased for those having major surgery or who have cancer. Reduced mobility or delayed discharge from hospital, for whatever reason, also increases the risk. Most OMFS patients are medically fit; their stay in hospital is frequently brief; even patients having orthognathic surgery or fixation of facial fractures may be admitted for only one or two nights. The main exceptions are those with multiple injuries and those receiving surgery for cancer.

Respiratory Complications

Smokers and those with pre-existing Chronic Obstructive Pulmonary Disease (COPD) are those who are at greatest risk of respiratory complications; anaesthetists can deal well with asthmatics.

During anaesthesia, there is a decrease in the action of the cilia lining the respiratory tract, causing a decrease in clearance of secretions. This, combined with the inability to cough and a decrease in ventilation, will lead to an accumulation of secretions, which may cause some obstruction and collapse of the peripheral airways called atelectasis. Atelectasis is most usually apparent as an early and transient mild pyrexia; it usually resolves. Resolution is aided by early mobilisation, breathing exercises and, if necessary, chest physiotherapy to clear mucous accumulation; nebulised bronchodilators may help. Resolution is compromised by the cigarette smoking, COPD, obesity and immobility.

If atelectasis does not resolve adequately, then the mucous accumulation will pre-dispose to secondary infection, often with nosocomial (hospital) organisms, i.e. pneumonia. The signs and symptoms may include pyrexia, cough, discoloured sputum on coughing, chest pain on breathing (pleuritic), tachypnoea, a dull note on percussion of the affected part of the chest accompanied by reduced breath sounds on auscultation of that part. Treatment may involve physiotherapy and breathing exercises, oxygen, and antibiotics against organisms cultured from the sputum. In severe cases, the patient may need ventilation.

A potential respiratory complication of OMFS is aspiration. The reason we see it so infrequently is because we take such care to avoid it. When operating on an anesthetised patient, the anaesthetist uses a cuffed endo-tracheal tube or laryngeal mask airway to prevent

Signs of Respiratory Complications
Pyrexia
Dyspnoea
Tachypnoea
Altered chest sounds

aspiration of saliva, blood, tooth or bone fragments etc., and we pack off the pharynx and use suction for the same purpose. Patients are only anaesthetised if they have been starved to reduce the risk of aspiration of stomach contents into the lungs; in an emergency, a naso-gastric tube will be passed by the anaesthetist to suction out stomach contents. Gastric acid can cause a chemical pneumonitis if it contaminates the lungs, which can produce a secondary infection and pneumonia.

Cardiovascular Complications

You may be called by a ward nurse to tell you that a patient has post-operative hypotension. This should be reported to your superior; some causes may be serious, but equally it can be benign. Patients may have a slightly low blood pressure because of medication such as ß-blockers or opiate analgesics given for pain. They may be slightly low on fluids and respond to having the end of the bed raised slightly or given some additional intra-venous fluid.

However, it is necessary to consider that the patient has shock, which is the term for inadequate tissue perfusion and oxygenation, leading to cellular damage and organ dysfunction. This is serious.

Hypovolemic shock, where there has been a large blood loss, is an unusual complication in our speciality, although it must be considered. It is unlikely that a large blood loss would go unnoticed as we are usually operating within the mouth and blood loss will be noticed. The patients must be assessed as a whole, particularly as young and fit patients have a high 'cardio-vascular reserve' and can compensate for a large blood loss before their pulse rate increases and blood pressure drops. Other signs of shock include a cold, clammy skin and poor capillary refill when squeezing an extremity. Shock will also produce a decrease in core body temperature, decreased urinary output and, in the case of hypovolemic shock, a decreased central venous pressure. All these are measured during major cancer surgery to monitor the consequence of blood loss.

The management of hypovolemic shock will be to resuscitate with a litre of crystalloid fluid (normal saline or dextrose saline followed by appropriate blood products; then find and arrest the bleeding. In the unlikely event you are first on the scene, you should 'peek and shriek', i.e. you should rapidly assess the situation and call for help. In most cases, the ward nurse will have realised the situation and already informed the intensive care out-reach team or the medical emergency team depending on the arrangements in your hospital.

Shock may result from inadequate cardiac output: cardiogenic shock. This may be caused by a myocardial infarct (MI), cardiac arrhythmias, or left ventricular failure (LVF) because of coronary artery disease,

previous MI or in elderly patients just from fluid overload. In most cases, the patient will be elderly, have a cardiac history and be taking cardiac medication. The patient should be assessed by examination of the cardiovascular system, looking for the signs of shock and ventricular failure. An ECG should be carried out and bloods tested for cardiac enzymes. This is a job for the medical emergency team or emergency physician on duty.

Occasionally you will see shock in an anaphylactic reaction; this should be managed as in the medical emergency chapter, with the medical emergency team being called as necessary.

Deep vein thrombosis (DVT) within the deep veins of the legs is a particular later complication of surgery that you should know about and hopefully will never see, as it is largely avoided though careful planning and prevention. After surgery, there may be a slight hypercoagulability, which may lead to a thrombosis in the deep veins of the leg. It is pre-disposed by immobility. Patients who are elderly, have cancer and have received major surgery are particularly at risk. The consequence may be varicose veins, but more

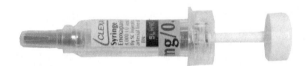

Enoxaparin (Clexane). 40 mg in a pre-filled syringe is a low molecular weight heparin usually given subcutaneously after surgery to help prevent DVT

Deep Vein Thrombosis Prevention
Pneumatic compression stockings
TED stockings
Low molecular weight heparin
Mobilise early

THROMBOPROHYLAXIS ASSESSMENT IS REQUIRED ON ADMISSION AND AT 24hrs

1

PROPHYLAXIS REQUIRED IF
☐ ONGOING REDUCED MOBILITY RELATIVE TO NORMAL STATE OR SURGICAL PATIENT

+ ONE OR MORE OF THE FOLLOWING RISK FACTORS

2 IF PROPHYLAXIS REQUIRED PRESCRIBE LMWH (OR SUITABLE ANTICOAGULANT) UNLESS CONTRA-INDICATED:

3 ALL AT RISK SURGICAL PATIENTS REQUIRE GRADUATED COMPRESSION STOCKINGS (GCS) AND / OR INTERMITTENT PNEUMATIC COMPRESSION (IPC) UNLESS CONTRA-INDICATED:

☐ Age > 60 ☐ Significantly reduced mobility for ≥ 3days ☐ BMI > 30kg/m² ☐ Active Cancer or Cancer treatment ☐ Previous PE / DVT ☐ Known thrombophilia / family history of DVT ☐ Significant medical comorbidity ☐ Acute illness / infection / inflammation ☐ Dehydration ☐ Surgical procedure, anaesthesia time > 60 mins ☐ Varicose veins with phlebitis ☐ Oestrogen therapy (HRT, OCP) ☐ Pregnant / post partum (see pregnancy booklet) ☐ No risk factors. No prophylaxis required.	**Contra-indications to LMWH/other anticoagulants** ☐ Active bleed (if intracranial liaise with consultant) ☐ On anticoagulants (caution with dual antiplatelets) ☐ Significant procedure related bleeding risk ☐ Acute stroke: haemorrhagic or large infarct ☐ Inherited bleeding disorder eg. haemophilia ☐ Severe / acute liver disease / caution if CrCl < 30ml/min ☐ Platelets < 75 or abnormal clotting screen ☐ BP > 230 systolic, or > 120 diastolic ☐ Lumbar puncture / epidural / spinal in previous 4 hours or within next 12 hours (for anticoagulants other than LMWH contact haematology SpR) ☐ Heparin induced thrombocytopenia ☐ None. Prescribe LMWH / other anticoagulant	**For medical patients in whom LMWH is ...** contraindicated consider GCS and / or IPC **Contra-indications to GCS** ☐ Peripheral arterial disease, suspected/proven ☐ Previous / planned revascularisation surgery ☐ Severe leg or pulmonary oedema ☐ Leg conditions worsened by stockings eg dermatitis, recent skin graft, gangrene, fragile skin, wounds, ulcers, cellulitis ☐ Major limb deformity / unusual leg shape or size ☐ Acute stroke ☐ Peripheral neuropathy / sensory impairment ☐ Allergy to GCS material ☐ None of the above. Prescribe GCS.
On admission Sign .... Date............. At 24 hrs and clinical situation change Sign .... Date.............	On admission Sign .... Date............. At 24 hrs and clinical situation change Sign .... Date.............	On admission Sign .... Date............. At 24 hrs and clinical situation change Sign .... Date.............

Thromboprophylaxis assessment form

particularly a breaking off of the clot to produce an embolus in the lung leading to right sided heart failure and death. Prevention starts at the pre-operative assessment, where all patients are considered for their risk. All hospitals have a thrombo-prophylaxis assessment checklist form used for all patients who are admitted and receive general anaesthesia.

Pneumatic compression of the calves during the operation prevents stasis within the veins of the legs. Thrombo-embolic deterrent (TED) stockings are worn by the patient while in hospital and low molecular weight heparin given after surgery to reduce the risk of clotting. You should know the risks of the individual patients on the wards with whose care you are assisting and double check they are getting the DVT prophylaxis they need.

DVT is usually silent with no physical signs, but there may be an oedematous swelling of the affected leg or pyrexia; this usually occurs 5 -7 days after surgery. A pulmonary embolus may present as chest pain, shortness of breath, tachypnoea, acute right sided heart failure or sudden death.

Urinary Complications

The principal urinary problems that you are likely to come across in OMFS patients are decreased urinary output (oliguria), urinary tract infection, and urinary retention.

Most of our patients are medically fit with normal renal function, so the most likely cause of oliguria is that the patient has inadequate fluid intake. In many of our major cases, particularly the long cancer cases which may involve significant blood loss, a urinary catheter will be placed in the operating theatre before surgery. Apart from the convenience of collecting urine when the patient is unconscious during surgery or in the post-operative period, it allows the output to be measured, which will help in calculating the fluid balance during surgery and beyond. Back on the ward, one would normally expect a normal patient to produce 1.5 litres of urine a day, i.e. about 60 ml. per hour; this will vary slightly. If several hours go by during which significantly less urine is produced, then something is wrong and in the absence of renal disease, it is most likely that they are 'dry' and need more fluid.

Where there is complete obstruction of urine output, then the urine will build up in the bladder and eventually the patient will be in pain and be distressed. The bladder will be distended and easily palpable above

Causes of Confusion
Hypoxia
Trauma
Drugs
Sepsis
Pain
Electrolyte imbalance
Dementia
Alcohol withdrawal

the pubis as a supra-pubic mass; palpation or pressure will be acutely uncomfortable or painful. If the patient has a catheter, then it will be blocked and should be flushed with saline or replaced. The most likely cause, however, will be benign hypertrophy of the prostate gland, which occurs commonly in elderly men. The patient will give a history of 'prostatic' symptoms indicating pre-existing outflow obstruction. These will include a poor stream on passing urine, hesitancy - delay in starting to micturate, dribbling - urine still leaking after stopping micturition, and a feeling that the bladder has not properly emptied after micturition. The patient with urinary retention will be pleased to have a urinary catheter passed as this will give immediate relief of the pain and discomfort. They should then be referred to a urologist.

Urinary catheters should be removed as soon as possible after their function is no longer needed; otherwise, they will act as a portal of infection into the urethra and bladder, leading to discomfort and pyrexia. Where patients have had them inserted in theatre for major cancer cases, they should be removed within a couple of days after surgery or as soon as measurement of urinary output is not needed. They should not be left in for the convenience of not having to help the patient to the bathroom. Apart from facilitating infection, a catheter will predispose to ulceration of the lining of the urethra and adhesions, leading to permanent urinary outflow obstruction. Patients' mobility is usually reduced by the presence and discomfort of a urinary catheter.

Post-Operative Confusion

Occasionally, a patient may become confused after surgery. The causes of confusion are many; these include hypoxia, trauma, medication, sepsis, pain, dementia, electrolyte imbalance and alcohol withdrawal.

A full physical examination should be carried out to exclude hypoxia or sepsis and a review made of all the medication that the patient is taking. A new or recent full blood count and biochemistry profile should be considered for a significant decrease in haemoglobin or change in electrolyte balance. Pain control should be reviewed and medication adjusted to get optimal relief.

Patients should have had their alcohol intake considered during their pre-operative assessment. Those who have a very high intake and who are deprived for several days can become very confused and disorientated with both auditory and visual hallucinations; this can be very distressing for all concerned. The problem can be prevented by administering a small but regular amount of alcohol to the patient in the form of a few ml. of whisky if necessary through a gastrostomy or naso-gastric tube.

Most frequently, confusion will be in an elderly patient with pre-existing dementia. Often an elderly patient will manage normally at home but when admitted to hospital to an unusually noisy environment and then given additional medication and some pain they may become completely disorientated, confused, uncooperative and uncontrollable. In these cases, assessment and management is best referred to a care of the elderly physician.

Pyrexia

All hospital inpatients have their temperature recorded regularly. Temperature can be measured in several ways, e.g. oral, rectal, vaginal. In the operating theatre during our major cancer cases, it is now usually measured within the bladder by a probe attached to a urinary catheter or by inserting a flexible rectal probe.

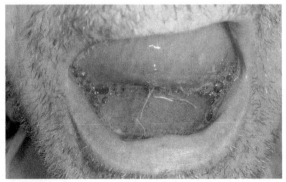

A radial forearm flap which has failed because the venous outflow has blocked. The patient will develop a severe pyrexia until the dead tissue is removed

Causes of Pyrexia
Early
Atelectasis
Blood transfusion
Intermediate
Infected catheters or lines
Tissue death
Chest infection
Late
All the above
Surgical wound infection
Venous thrombosis

On the ward, however, the most popular way is tympanic temperature using a probe placed into an ear; this is both quick and hygienic.

Normally, temperature will vary at different times of the day, menstrual cycle, ambient room temperature, clothing and after food or drink. It is therefore not the absolute temperature we are concerned about as much as the variation in the particular patient. The temperature will vary around 37.5°C.

In the immediate post-operative period, the most common causes of pyrexia will be atelectasis, as discussed above, or blood transfusion. Transfused blood is always matched for compatibility with the ABO and Rhesus systems. However, there will be other antibodies which will cause a reaction in the host and hence a mild pyrexia.

In the intermediate period 3 to 5 days post-op a pyrexia is likely to be caused by infection, particularly of in-dwelling catheters such as urinary catheters, central venous lines and peripheral venous lines. If the patient develops a wound infection at the site of operation, it is unlikely to have developed enough to cause a rise in temperature by this stage. However, tissue death, such as a tissue flap used to reconstruct a defect caused during cancer resection, may well cause pyrexia if it is starting to lose vitality. You should check all the sites of lines and catheters for signs of inflammation, the operation site, and report the pyrexia and your findings for your superior to review. You should also examine the chest in case atelectasis is developing into a chest infection.

A late pyrexia may be due to any of the above causes, but In addition, an infection at the operative site must be more seriously considered together with venous thrombosis.

Recognition of critical illness

Besides recognising complications, it is desirable that you should understand how to recognise someone who is 'going off' after surgery, i.e. becoming critically ill. However, it is likely to be the ward nurse who raises the alarm. The nurse may alert the intensive care outreach team, who will send one of their specialist nurses to assess the problem. The system will be different between hospitals; in some it may the medical emergency team who is alerted; in others it may be you who is called, in which case you should make a brief assessment but not delay passing the problem up the chain of command.

The onset of complications can often be followed by the nurses' observation records which used to be kept on a chart at the end of the patient's bed but now are more likely to be recorded onto a mobile phone at the patient's bedside and transferred to a computer record which will be visible to all the staff. The computer will work out the MEWS (modified early warning) score and a referral to the acute care practitioner, intensive care outreach team, medical emergency team or high dependency unit will be triggered by a score of 5 or more. MEWS scoring detects when a patient is becoming seriously ill at an early stage so that there can be early intervention.

The routine 'obs' includes blood pressure, pulse rate, respiratory rate, temperature, oxygen saturation level of consciousness, and pain score (from 1 to 3). After major surgery, such as a head and neck cancer resection and reconstruction, the patient will also have a fluid input and output chart; urine output measurement will be possible because of a urinary catheter.

The onset of problems will be predicted by a rising MEWS score. A patient's temperature or pulse rate may be consistently raised or their oxygen saturation decreased. Decrease in blood pressure is often a late change in hypovolaemia due to physiological compensation; it should always be treated seriously. A decrease in urine output is potentially a bad sign.

The most significant observational signs to indicate critical illness are the respiratory rate and pulse with blood pressure. The normal respiratory rate should be between 12 and 20 per minute. If this rate is higher than this or is increasing, this is a significant sign that all is not well. If the pulse rate is above the systolic blood pressure, this too is serious and requires immediate medical attention. This is known as the 'Portsmouth' sign.

8. Surgical Instruments

Instruments are supplied in trays double wrapped and autoclaved. Bench top sterilisers, such as those frequently used in dental practices, are not used in hospitals because of their unreliability and the need for vigorous and documented daily testing and servicing. Some instruments which are infrequently used will be packed singly, and some will be single use and disposable.

The nurses in the operating theatre will keep a record of which trays and individual instruments are needed by particular surgeons for particular operations. For surgery in the outpatient setting, there are minor oral surgery sets, which contain basic instruments for exodontia, and soft tissue sets, which contain the fewer instruments needed for biopsies and skin surgery. In the operating theatre there will be oral surgery sets, facial trauma, osteotomy, plating sets and 'wiring of jaw' sets which are nowadays infrequently used.

Each sterile tray sits on disinfected stainless steel wheeled trolleys. The infrequently used instruments will be double wrapped and designed for a nurse to open the outer layer and drop the instrument wrapped within an inner layer onto the sterile tray already opened.

In the operating theatre, there will always be a 'scrub nurse' who will pass the instruments to the surgeon as they are needed. For minor ops in the clinic, the surgeon will help themselves from the instrument tray. After use, the instruments are sent back to the sterile supply department in the trays or baskets they have been used from. Some items cannot be cleaned adequately prior to sterilisation so should be treated as single use; surgical burs fall into this category. Before being returned, gross contamination should be removed from instruments whilst wearing kitchen gloves.

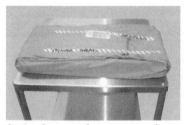

1. A minor oral surgery set is on the surgical trolley for use in the clinic. The first layer of the drape is opened with clean hands touching only the outside and is allowed to drop back around the trolley

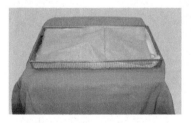

2. The tray contains sterile (green) drapes to cover the patient, in this case for minor oral surgery. One goes behind the patient's head and the other over them

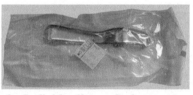

3. Individually packed retractor. The wrapping is designed to be peeled open and dropped onto a sterile tray

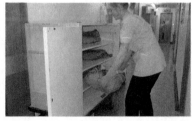

4. Dirty instruments are returned for processing in wheeled strong metal trolleys

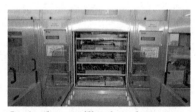

5. At the sterilisation department the trays of instruments are put into the washer/disinfector machine. The instruments are mechanically cleaned with jets of water at 90°C in an alkaline detergent, then dried

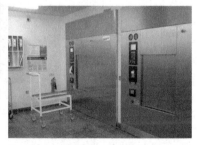

6. Then autoclaved. This vacuum autoclave draws all the air out and then injects steam under pressure. It repeats this alternately four times and on the last occasion it holds the steam in at between 134 and 137° for 3 to 3½ minutes at 2 bar pressure. The trays are then dried. The whole cycle takes 45 minutes

9. Tracheostomy in Oral and Maxillofacial Surgery

A tracheostomy, where a tube is inserted through the skin of the anterior neck directly into the trachea, is used routinely in OMFS to facilitate breathing or ventilation of the lungs. We use the technique principally in major cancer cases where the surgery itself, or bleeding or swelling afterwards, might obstruct the airway. It thus makes the process safer and reduces risk. It will also facilitate providing a second anaesthetic in the post-operative period if something should go wrong, such as bleeding or reconstruction flap failure. The second use in OMFS is in major facial trauma, where there may be multiple fractures of the mandible, tongue swelling or fragments of broken tooth or bleeding which might compromise the airway.

There are other indications for tracheostomy, such as maintenance of the airway in patients who have reduced consciousness or who need longer term artificial ventilation of the lungs in an intensive care unit. We carry out tracheostomy by open operation with a patient under general anaesthesia, but in intensive care units it may be performed using a percutaneous technique by the intensive care physicians.

Tracheostomy care

Following tracheostomy, the two main concerns are that the tube might block or become displaced. The patient should therefore be looked after by nurses who are skilled in the monitoring of patients with tracheostomy. There should be regular inspections of the tracheostomy tube with regular, 4 hourly removal and cleaning of the inner tube.

During normal breathing, inspired air is warmed and humidified in the nasal passages. A tracheostomy bypasses the nose and if inspired air is not humidified, normal cilia function in the airways is reduced and there can be an accumulation of thick sputum which can block the tracheostomy tube. To humidify inspired air a heated water based unit may be used for those being ventilated or using high oxygen or for ambulant patients breathing unaided a bib may be worn which is a layer of foam which absorbs moister from expired air and makes it available for inspiration or a heat moister exchanger can be placed at the end of the tube. This comprises a metal gauze, foam or a condenser element impregnated with a hydroscopic compound which conserves heat and moisture on expiration and recycles it during inspiration. Where the patient is producing thick mucous, they can be given a saline nebuliser to loosen this all up.

Tracheostomy

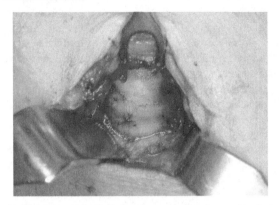

1. Under endo-tracheal anaesthesia patient is positioned with neck extended. Trachea is exposed thorough horizontal incision.

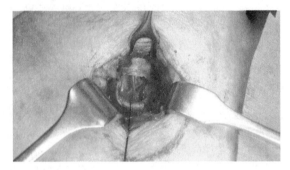

2. A window is cut in trachea at level of 2nd & 3rd tracheal ring. The anaesthetic tube is seen within.

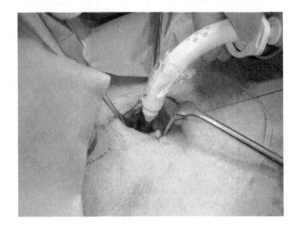

3. The anaesthetist withdraws the endotracheal tube as the tracheostomy tube is introduced.

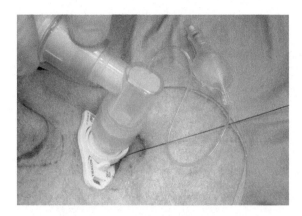

4. The anaesthetic circuit is attached to the tube, the cuff is inflated and the tube is secured to the patient with sutures and/or tape around the neck.

The tracheostomy tube should be sucked out with a suction catheter for no longer than 15 seconds every four hours and the inner tracheotomy cannula removed for cleaning.

An equipment trolley should be available on the ward to deal with tracheostomy emergencies (blockage or displacement); it is often kept in a 'tracheostomy box' containing tracheostomy tubes, tracheal dilators, inner tubes, tapes, etc. This should be kept close to the patient in case of emergency and move with them if they are moved.

The tube should be securely fixed to the patient by sutures or tape around the neck; this should be checked regularly. The whole tracheostomy tube should be changed every 7 to 10 days. In most of our patients, the tube will not be needed after a few days post-operation.

Tracheostomy removal

It is desirable that the tracheostomy be removed as soon as it is not needed. The air should be removed from the cuff and the tube should be suctioned to remove secretions which might have accumulated above the cuff. Before removing the tube, it is essential that the patient can breathe around the tube, which may be facilitated by using a fenestrated tube. The tube can be blocked off for a while so that we can be confident that the patient no longer needs it. The speech and language therapist can be consulted as they have expertise in airway patency. Tube removal is best carried out first thing on a weekday morning, ensuring there are sufficient trained staff available to deal with any problems.

Outer tracheostomy cannula

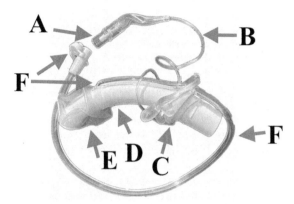

A: *Air introduction port* B: *Air connecting tube to cuff* C: *Flange* D: *Outer Cannula shaft* E: *Air cuff* F: *Sub-glottic port and suction line to aspirate secretions from the trachea*

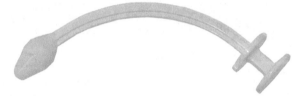

Introducer: *Is placed inside outer tube when tube is inserted into trachea at operation.*

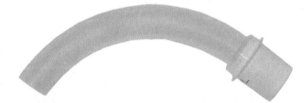

Inner cannula: Locks in place in outer tube & can be removed for cleaning.

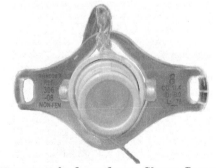

Outer cannula from front: Shows flange marked with size, cuff air tube, sub-glottis suction line and attachments for tape to secure around neck

10. <u>Minor Oral Surgery</u>

We will now introduce you to a minor oral surgery (MOS) procedure to show the process. A biopsy of a white patch in the floor of mouth is to be performed, assisted by a staff nurse. Biopsies are often carried out on a biopsy clinic with the surgeon and just one nurse assisting. For surgical procedures involving dental extractions, which may need a drill, or for laser surgery, the surgeon is assisted by two nurses, a 'scrub nurse' and a 'runner'. The scrub nurse assists while the runner remains unsterile and fetches equipment, sets up the drill and suction or programs the laser; just as in the operating theatre.

Always check a patient's name, hospital number, address and date of birth before operating. Never have a second set of notes on a surface with the notes of the patient you are dealing with and never label specimen pots or request forms before they are used. These can all lead to mistakes.

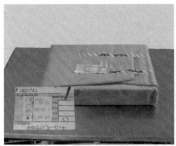

1. Instruments arrive from ASDU (Area Sterilising & Disinfection Unit) or CSSD (Central Sterile Services Department) wrapped in paper and closed with autoclave tape. Each has a label (inset) which identifies the instruments . This is placed in the patient's notes so the instruments can be traced should there be any contamination issue later.

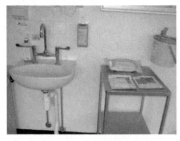

2. The room must have a wash basin with taps that can be elbow operated, surgical scrub, a flat surface for the surgical gown and gloves, and a sharps disposal bin.

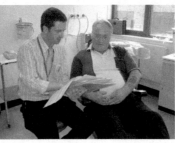

3. The patient is identified by checking their name, address and date of birth against the notes. The patient should already have given informed consent for the procedure.

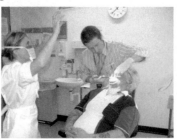

4. Local anaesthetic is administered by the surgeon wearing non sterile examination gloves.

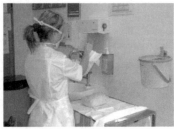

5. Meanwhile the nurse, who is wearing a plastic disposable apron (cheap), scrubs and dons sterile gloves.

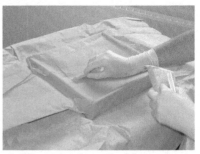

6. The tray of surgical instruments is already on a clean surgical trolley. The outer blue covering has been opened with clean hands from the outside. Now the inner sterile green layer is opened by the nurse wearing sterile gloves.

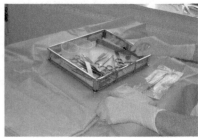

7. The pack contains the instruments and sterile towels to drape the patient.

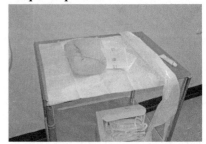

8. The sterile gown for the surgeon has been opened on to a sterile towel with the gloves.

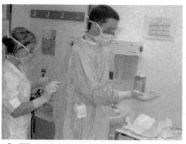

9. The surgeon scrubs, dons gown & gloves, while the nurse ties up from behind. The surgeon's gown is sterile, the ties are behind so may be tied with or without sterile gloves.

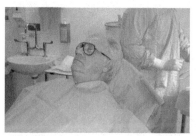

10. The patient is covered by a sterile gown from the tray with another behind his head. He wears protective wide lens safety spectacles.

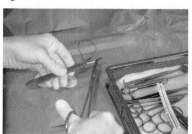

11. The blade is placed on the handle (unless a disposable scalpel is used) and the suture mounted on the needle holder.

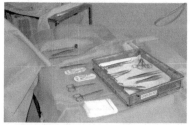

12. Instruments most likely to be used have been laid out of the tray with sutures and swabs.

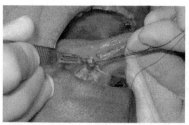

13. The procedure is carried out by the surgeon who helps himself to instruments from the tray and is assisted by the nurse.

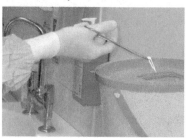

14. When finished, the surgeon disposes of the blade, suture and needle into the sharps bin.

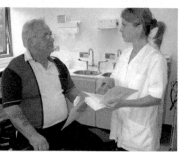

15 While the surgeon writes up the operation note the nurse goes through the post-operative instruction leaflet with the patient.

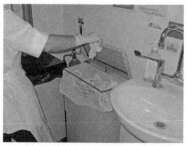

16. Contaminated disposables, like gloves, swabs etc, are placed into a yellow clinical waste bag. Uncontaminated material is placed in a black household waste bag (cheaper to dispose of).

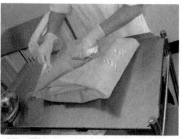

17. The used instruments are wrapped up.

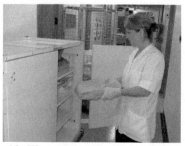

18. The wrapped instruments are placed into the contaminated instruments trolley which is returned to the sterile supply department at the end of the day.

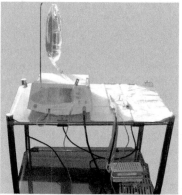

Where surgery requires the use of a drill, suction or laser this will need to be set up before the patient enters the room. A third person should be present to act as 'runner', to fetch and carry things. The drill unit is set up on a trolley with the end of the cord covered with a sterile plastic sheath. Fluid from an IV bag passes to the hand piece through a sterile tube. The drill unit is operated with a foot control which simultaneously pumps the fluid to the bur

11. <u>Sharps Injuries and the Blood Borne Viruses</u>

All clinical workers in dental surgery are at risk of needle stick (inoculation) injury. The greatest risk is from the penetration of the operator's or assistant's skin with a hollow bore needle contaminated with blood (or saliva). However, the skin can be penetrated by anything sharp, which includes any sharp instrument, wire, broken glass, sharp tooth or even bone. Also included is contamination of the operator's skin at the site of a cut or abrasion or the contamination of mucous membrane of the mouth or eye.

The definition of 'exposure-prone procedures' includes nearly all of clinical dentistry. Surgeons or nurses in training, including dental, are at the highest risk, so it is wise to know as much about this hazard and how to reduce the risks before you start. It has been estimated that about 80 % of injuries are preventable.

The risk is not limited to just hepatitis B, C and HIV. There is also a risk from human T-lymphotropic retroviruses, hepatitis D and G virus, cytomegalovirus, Epstein Barr Virus, parvovirus, transfusion-transmitted virus, West Nile Virus, malarial parasites and prion agents, which may cause spongiform encephalopathies.

Although Hepatitis B is the most infectious, the good news is that if you have been immunised and you are one of the 90% who respond with a good antibody level, then your risk should be zero. If you have not responded to immunisation (usually obese men first immunised at over 40 years of age) then the risk of seroconverting can be reduced with post exposure prophylaxis with immunoglobulin.

Least infectious is HIV. The risk can be reduced by use of post exposure prophylaxis. There have been few proven cases of transmission to health care workers and these are mostly where the worker has received a deep wound with a hollow needle used for taking blood from an infected patient in the latter stage of the disease when they have a high viral load. As with all blood borne virus transmission, the risk of mucous membrane contamination is much less than with a skin puncture wound. Although prevalence of hepatitis C in the UK is only about 0.02 % of the population, the seroconversion rate from accidental inoculation from a Hepatitis C carrier is greater than that of HIV.

What to do when you sustain a sharps injury when operating

You should stop operating, un-scrub and remove gloves and wash the injured part thoroughly with soap and running water. Bleeding should be encouraged. If

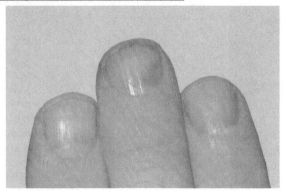

Blood on fingers after an orthognathic operation. Blood borne viruses will not penetrate intact skin but they will if the skin is damaged. There is a high risk of glove puncture when using wires and operating where there are fixed orthodontic appliances such as in orthognathic surgery. Wear double gloves.

your eye, mouth or nose have been splashed with blood or blood contaminated saliva, they should be washed with copious amounts of running water. The on duty manager or your superior should be informed.

Your employer will have a policy and procedure to follow which should be available in the operating theatre, outpatient clinic and on the hospital intranet. The incident should be reported to the Occupational Health Department. There will almost certainly be a form to be filled in. If it is closed, there will probably be an on-call nurse or the service will be provided by the Emergency Department.

The patient (donor)

The patient (if identified) should be told of the mishap and reassured that there is negligible risk to them. A risk assessment of the patient for the blood-borne viruses should be made from previous history and habits. This, again, will probably involve a form. A blood sample should be taken for HIV antibodies, hepatitis B surface antigen and hepatitis C. Of course, the patient must give consent for this, but in practice this is seldom refused. The patient's serum will be tested as soon as possible.

The health worker (recipient)

The requirement for specific prophylactic treatment will be determined by the Occupational Health Department or whoever is on call for it, from initial risk assessment and the immune status of the staff member for Hepatitis B. If the initial assessment reveals negligible risk then no action is needed, but if there is a significant risk then the health worker should have baseline blood tests for HIV and hepatitis C antibody and post exposure prophylaxis should be prescribed which should be started immediately.

How to avoid sharps injuries

1. Wear gloves for all clinical procedures where hands might be contaminated with blood or saliva

2. Cover cuts or skin abrasions with a waterproof dressing before donning gloves

3. Never re-sheath needles. Remove needles from syringes and blades from knives with forceps and always away from you

4. When carrying out minor oral surgery with an assistant, but no scrub nurse, the surgeon should dispose of sharps into the sharps bin at the end to avoid risk to the nursing staff. The sharps bin should be disposed of when ¾ full

5. In theatre the scrub nurse places all sharps on a sharps pad which is sealed and placed in the sharps bin

6. Surgical knives should be passed between scrub nurse and surgeon in a bowl

7. During surgery retract with instruments not hands

8. Double glove for high risk procedures such as placing wire around teeth. This does not avoid the risk of skin puncture but may reduce the volume inoculated if this happens

9. Change gloves if punctured. Indicator gloves worn as an inside layer may show up a puncture

10. Wear large rim spectacles or a mask to prevent eye contamination when operating. There is a small risk of seroconverting from blood or saliva splashed into the eye. There is no risk from contamination of intact skin

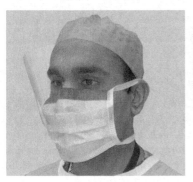

A face mask incorporating eye protection. This is cumbersome; you may prefer wide rimmed glasses.

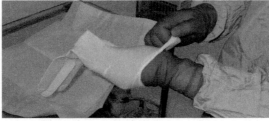

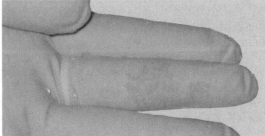

For high risk procedures such as when using wires 'indicator' gloves can be worn beneath normal gloves. If outer glove is penetrated moisture will show green.

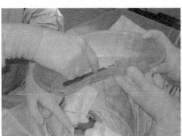

Scrub nurse passes knife to surgeon in a dish.

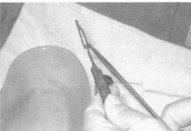

Blades are removed with a needle holder (centre) and placed on a sharps pad which is sealed before disposal (right). A disposable scalpel is even safer

12. <u>Being on Call, Accidents and Emergencies</u>

The Emergency Medicine Department, until recently known as Accident and Emergency (and may still be in some hospitals) exists to treat patients who need immediate attention.

Some patients who are seriously ill or injured may arrive by ambulance or helicopter (ambucopter) and may, if their lives are in danger, be transferred to the resuscitation room (resus). However, most will be 'walking wounded' and will be seen initially by a triage nurse who will make an initial assessment, decide the priority of their problems and sometimes start treatment. Patients with minor ailments may be given advice and sent on their way to see their GP the next day. After seeing the nurse, the patients will either be seen by an emergency medicine doctor and managed by them or referred to specialist services; this maybe you.

Among the patients you will be asked to see, there will inevitably be some with major multiple injuries, which will include facial injuries. However, most of the patients to be managed by OMFS will walk in. These will include soft tissue lacerations from fights and falls, dental injuries, dog bites to the face (particularly in children), and facial fractures, mostly from interpersonal violence.

Initial assessment

When you first encounter an urgent patient, like all clinical encounters with patients, you should have an order in your mind how you are going to go about things. Traditionally, doctors have relied on firstly taking a history before examining the patient and then ordering special tests. This still seems to be the safest way of proceeding. If you follow a sequence with clear

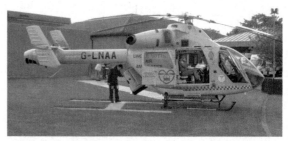
Although some patients will be brought in by ambulance and a few by ambucopter the majority you see will be walking wounded.

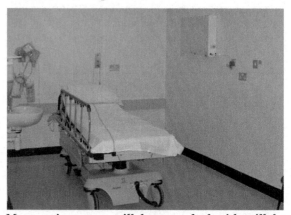
Most patients you will have to deal with will be presented to you on a trolley in a treatment cubicle. You should attempt to deal with the patient as swiftly as possible and if suturing is likely to be prolonged move them to the ward or outpatient clinic.

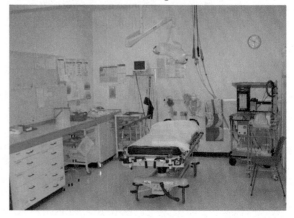
Those with serious injuries are brought from the ambulance on a trolley straight to the resuscitation room. This contains anaesthetic and other equipment for resuscitation.

OMFS cases in Emergency Medicine

Facial Trauma

    Facial lacerations
    Jaw fractures
    Malar fractures
    Dental Injuries
    Polytrauma including facial injuries

Dental Sepsis

Bleeding from the mouth

Dislocated Jaws

---

headings in your mind, you will reduce the risk of missing anything.

Clinical records written in the Emergency Department are those most likely to be referred to later, often for the purpose of insurance or legal claims or police statements. It is vitally important that your notes are legible and comprehensive. The date and time you saw the patient must be clearly written; this should include the year.

There will be many occasions when you will be the first called upon to diagnose fractures of the facial skeleton. After a short while, the common patterns of injury will become obvious to you and the task will become easy. Except in a very few unusual cases of severe haemorrhage, bony facial injuries are not life threatening and can be dealt with at a leisurely pace.

Most injuries will be to the mandible and zygoma. In some cases, the patient can be discharged home with analgesics and asked to attend the outpatient clinic for assessment. However, most with mandibular fractures will need to be admitted to hospital for operation, usually within 24 hours. They should have a cannula placed and intra-venous fluids and antibiotics started. If the patient has a very displaced mandibular fracture, a bridle wire may be applied around teeth next to the fracture to partly reduce it. This will help prevent movement and hence minimise pain and swelling.

Some patients will have multiple injuries. Except where there is airway obstruction or uncontrolled bleeding, the facial injuries should be treated after orthopaedic or abdominal injuries, as these can be life threatening. The emergency medicine doctor will have made an initial assessment. If the patient has soft tissue facial lacerations and/or loose or badly damaged teeth, it may be appropriate to operate on these at the same time if the patient is being taken to the operating theatre for other injuries. Definitive management of facial fractures is best deferred until better imaging and consent is obtained. The second on-call should always be informed when a patient presents to you, so that an appropriate assessment can be made, appropriate notes

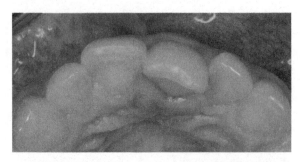

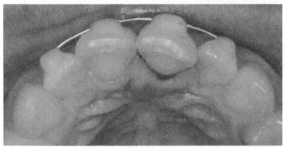

A displaced (luxated)incisor repositioned and splinted with orthodontic wire attached with acid etched composite.
See the technique at: https://vimeo.com/137957560

written, and the management of the face planned in context with other injuries.

You will soon become confident about which patients should be admitted to a surgical ward and which can come back to an outpatient clinic for follow up or assessment. You will need to know in advance which are the best clinic days to bring patients back to so you can tell them.

Dental trauma

Teeth that have been displaced (luxated) should be reduced into their correct position and splinted to adjacent teeth. This is best achieved with stainless steel orthodontic wire attached by acid etch composite for 4 weeks. The aim is to secure the teeth, but not so rigidly that there is no physiological movement within the periodontal ligament. A rigidly splinted tooth has a higher risk of becoming ankylosed in the bone and of resorbing later. Our preferred method in the emergency department is to splint the teeth with thermoplastic special tray plastic or a temporary crown material and bring the patient back to the outpatient clinic in working hours and make a splint using orthodontic wire attached using an acid etch technique.

Teeth that have been traumatised but not displaced (concussed) need no active splinting and where the tooth is loosened but not displaced (subluxed) splinting may be placed for 2 weeks to decrease discomfort in function. Teeth that have been completely avulsed can be washed gently with water or saline, without touching the root, re-implanted and splinted with wire for 4 weeks.

An emergency department may not stock the instruments or materials you will need to give first aid for dental injuries or to suture and pack bleeding extraction sockets. We keep these in a toolbox which our surgeons can carry to where they might be needed; it is kept stocked by a staff nurse. Most departments will have similar arrangements. We suggest you find out where you may find instruments and familiarise yourself with them before you see patients.

Admitting a patient with a facial fracture

Many patients presenting with facial fractures will require hospital admission, but not quite all. Some surgeons may prefer to operate upon fractures of the malar complex (zygoma) at a later stage when the swelling has gone down and so the patient will not need admission. As long as they have been cleared from having any head injury and their eyes are uninjured, they can be discharged home with an appointment to be reviewed in the outpatient clinic by the consultant at a convenient time. In busy units with a high trauma load, there may be regular dedicated trauma clinics for this purpose. The same applies to unilateral mandibular condyle, orbital blow out and isolated nasal fractures.

It will also be necessary for you to arrange for patients to be reviewed who have sustained facial trauma but not any obvious fracture or soft tissue injury. You may soon become proficient at examining patients and interpreting facial x-ray and CT images, but the consultant will be better so it is wise that he or she checks to make sure you have not missed something.

The standard management for mandibular fractures is open reduction and fixation with titanium plates, which should preferably be done within 24 hours of injury. Once you have made the diagnosis, inform your consultant or specialist registrar so they can see the patient. A ward bed should be found (which should not be your job) and the patient admitted. Accurate notes should be made as described in the chapter on examination of the injured face and the patient and any accompanying friends or relatives made aware of what the plan is.

Facial Fractures Some Key Points

• No admission required for zygomatic, unilateral mandibular condylar or isolated nasal fractures with no head or eye injury

• Check facial imaging with your 2nd on call or supervisor to ensure no undiagnosed fractures

• All other mandibular fractures require hospital admission – contact your superior and inform bed manager

• All mandibular fractures (except isolated condylar) are compound into the mouth – prescribe antibiotics, 'nil by mouth', IV infusion and plan for surgery

• All maxillary (midface) fractures require hospital admission – high impact force - clear neck injury with trauma or orthopaedic team

• Severe facial injuries can compromise airway – significant bleeding and soft tissue injuries, loose teeth or foreign bodies – immediate surgery

Having arranged with your superior of when and where surgery is to take place, the operating theatre and anaesthetist should be informed. The anaesthetist will want to know of the patient's general health and if they can open their mouth easily, as this will have a bearing on the anaesthetic (see anaesthetic chapter).

All mandibular fractures (apart from condylar) are compound into the mouth so it is normal practice for the patients to be prescribed antibiotics to reduce the risk of infection which is heightened because a foreign body (titanium plate) is going to be placed into the fracture. The patient will need to be 'nil by mouth' because they will have a general anaesthetic and so will need an IV infusion to give them fluids and the antibiotics will be given IV as well, usually co-amoxiclav. 2½ litres of fluid should be prescribed on a fluid chart to run over 24 hours and if the patient has been drinking alcohol they will already be a little dehydrated so the quantity should be increased (see the prescribing fluids chapter).

All patients with mid-face maxillary fractures will need hospital admission. These fractures require a substantial force to produce, so you should assume the patient has a head injury associated with it and that there might be a neck injury as well. The neck should be imaged and cleared by an orthopaedic surgeon or trauma team before the neck is moved substantially without the patient wearing a neck collar to protect it.

Although most facial injuries are not life threatening in some severe injuries, there may be significant bleeding, loose teeth or associated soft tissue injuries, which may compromise the airway. In these cases, the first contact with the patient may be in the resuscitation room where there will be an anaesthetist who has already sedated and intubated the patient. In this scenario, they will want a tracheostomy to ensure no airway obstruction. The surgeon will usually operate straight away to do the tracheostomy, remove severely damaged or loose teeth, and arrest haemorrhage.

Admitting a patient with dental sepsis

Many patients attend emergency departments with dental pain. It is not the duty of the hospital or OMFS department to relieve the primary care dental services of the pleasure or responsibility of relieving pain. However, among these patients will be a number who have an abscess with pus formation, which could cause systemic illness or even loss of life eventually should it progress unchecked.

Patients with apical periodontitis or small abscesses can be advised to seek urgent care from a primary dentist the next day or, if deteriorating, from your own out-patient clinic the next day.

Indications for hospital admission for dental sepsis

Firm extra-oral swelling (not just soft oedema)

Limitation of mouth opening

Difficulty swallowing

Swelling down to the neck

Swelling up to the eye

Pyrexia

Systemically unwell

Dental sepsis investigations

OPG radiograph

Full blood count (? Raised white count)

Glucose (? Undiagnosed diabetic)

Urea and electrolytes

Dental sepsis immediate management

Inform registrar or consultant

IV line and fluids

IV antibiotics (usually co-amoxiclav or metronidazole)

Analgesia (IV paracetamol if oral is inadequate)

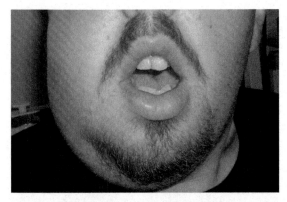

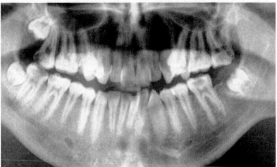

Patient with pain at LR7 presented to dentist who couldn't be bothered to remove the tooth and instead prescribed two antibiotics over two weeks. Now he has trismus and extra-oral swelling and needs admission for removal of the tooth and extra-oral drainage. Such negligence is commonplace.

Some patients with advanced abscesses will need hospital admission for removal of the causative tooth and drainage of pus. Most of the patients who have progressed to this state will have been seen in a primary care facility and inadequately been prescribed antibiotics, often over several weeks. Sometimes they may have been seen by a medical practitioner who cannot do anything more to help, but more usually they have seen a dentist who simply cannot be bothered to remove or drain the tooth properly.

Full notes should be made, which should include a dental assessment and a pan-oral X-ray image requested. A raised temperature indicates systemic upset. Where there is undrained pus present, the temperature will be 'swinging' up and down. The temperature should be taken every six hours, it will be done routinely by the ward nurses as part of the normal 'observations'. Once the pus is drained, it should dip and stay down.

Occasionally, a previously undiagnosed diabetic may present with severe dental sepsis because of being immunocompromised by their condition; we therefore always check their glucose. A full blood count may show an increased white cell count depending upon the systemic upset caused by the abscess. A sample for biochemistry urea and electrolytes should be taken.

Once on the ward, the patient should have an IV drip; if they are pyrexial, they will have an increased insensible loss of fluid so will need more than the standard 2½ litres over 24 hours. They may be dehydrated if they have not been eating and drinking normally because of pain or swelling.

For a patient who is unwell enough to need hospital admission, an antibiotic is appropriate but is not the definitive treatment. A broad-spectrum antibiotic active against the gram-negative organisms which are normally present should be given intravenously. This would normally be co-amoxiclav or metronidazole. The antibiotic has the effect of limiting the spread of pus through the soft tissues so it becomes localised and therefore easier to drain surgically. The patient will also need analgesia.

In most cases, 24 hours of IV antibiotics will localise the swelling and then the causative tooth should be removed and pus drained. If the patient can open their mouth sufficiently, the tooth can be removed and pus drained with local anaesthetic. However, most cases will need to be done in the operating theatre; the anaesthetist will need to know about limited mouth opening so that someone skilled in dealing with this can be involved (see anaesthetic chapter).

When the tooth is removed and pus drained, a swab of pus is usually sent to the laboratory for culture and antibiotic sensitivity. However, we have found this rarely affects the patient's management as once the pus is drained, they improve and usually don't require more antibiotics. It is normal practice to change the antibiotics to oral administration at this stage rather than stop them altogether and to stop them completely when the patient goes home in a day or two. If an extra-oral incision has been made to drain the pus, we normally sew in a plastic drain to facilitate drainage and prevent the skin from healing over the pus; this is normally secured to the skin with one or two silk sutures.

If the patient has a very neglected mouth, it may be appropriate to remove all teeth that are beyond restoration under the same anaesthetic. However, it may not be in the patient's best interest to cause the increased bleeding this will involve if their trismus is severe, and the anaesthetist and operating theatre staff may not be happy for you to spend over an hour doing a difficult full or part dental clearance if there are other cases waiting for time on an 'emergency' operating list.

After extraction of the cause of dental sepsis and drainage of pus, it is to be expected that the patient will become apyrexial and well although oedematous swelling will take some days to resolve.

A small minority of patients may have overwhelming sepsis and pyrexia despite extraction and attempted drainage of pus. In these cases, the patient may remain unwell and pyrexia will continue.

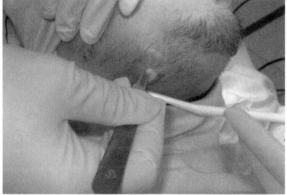

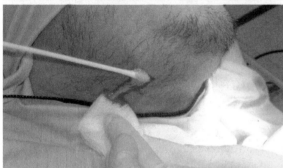

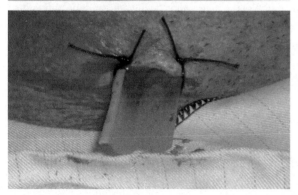

After incision and drainage a swab is usually taken for microbiology culture and sensitivity and a drain sewed in to facilitate drainage of pus.

Sometimes, ultrasound, CT or MRI imaging may be needed to locate pockets of concealed pus, and a microbiologist may be contacted for advice. Blood samples may be needed for cultures and antibiotic sensitivity, samples are taken at the peak of a 'swinging' pyrexia when it is expected organisms may be released into the circulation. Other markers of inflammation, such as C-reactive protein (CRP) are of little use in dental sepsis. Such overwhelming sepsis is rare from a dental cause.

Once the patient can eat and drink sufficient calories and fluid and they can care for themselves, they may be discharged home. They do not need to stay in hospital until all the pus has drained out; they can be given dressings to take home to mop up draining pus, and the district nurses can be called upon to help with this. It is usual to remove drains before the patient is discharged but not essential; they can return to the out-patient clinic for this. Remember, early discharge from hospital is desirable for other patients as pus on the ward is an infection risk to everybody.

A review of the patient in the clinic is needed after treatment of an extensive abscess in order to access extra-oral wound healing and for the rare occasions of recurrent infection.

Dental Sepsis Key Points

● Dental pain – provide sympathy and ibuprofen

● Patients with advanced abscesses – hospital admission – removal of causative tooth and drainage of pus – intra-oral and/or extra-oral

● Adverse signs requiring hospital admission – firm facial swelling, trismus, difficulty in swallowing, swelling extending to neck or eye

● Full history and examination, OPG image, check patient's temperature, blood tests including glucose, intravenous drip, antibiotics, anaesthetic assessment, drainage in operating theatre

● Extra oral drainage requires securing a plastic drain to the skin with sutures

● Change IV to oral antibiotics after successful drainage of pus

● It is optional to remove all other unrestorable teeth

● Remove drain before discharging patient even though some wounds may continue to discharge

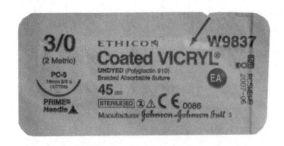

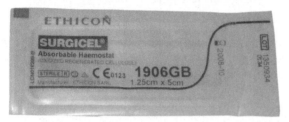

Bleeding after dental extraction is usually stopped by pressure from biting on a gauze swab for 20 minutes followed by packing the socket with oxidized cellulose gauze (Surgicel) and suturing with 3/0 Vicryl. Tranexamic acid given intravenously is wonderful for difficult cases.

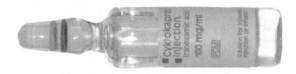

Dealing with Bleeding from the Mouth

Sometimes patients will present with haemorrhage after dental extraction performed outside of the hospital. The patient may present to the hospital either of their own volition or because the dentist who carried out the extraction has not been contactable. Patients who are bleeding must be seen and treated. Suturing the sockets and packing them with oxidised cellulose gauze is usually effective, but sometimes haemorrhage can be persistent and require hospital admission.

When you arrive, you will probably find that the patient is biting on a gauze swab or spitting blood and saliva into a kidney bowl they have been given for the purpose; the bowl may contain many blood stained swabs and the patient may be distressed.

At first, you should sit the patient comfortably and not quite horizontal on a treatment trolley with a good light and suction. Decontaminate your hands and place on personal protective equipment and gloves. Suck out the patient's mouth to observe where the bleeding is

coming from and get them to bite on a tightly folded swab for 15 minutes.

You should then take a full history which should include how long they have been bleeding for, where the surgery was carried out and what was done, whether they were given any instructions, if they have been rinsing their mouth, etc. A medical history is mandatory, including any previous surgery and associated bleeding, bruising or abnormal bleeding if they cut themselves. Enquire about their medical status. Bleeding can result from liver disease caused by alcohol abuse, hepatitis or cancer, bone marrow disease from cancer, such as leukaemia or recent cancer chemotherapy. Platelet function can be compromised by renal disease or auto-immune thrombocytopenia.

There are many drugs which may contribute towards haemorrhage, including aspirin and dipyridamole. If the patient is taking the anti-coagulant warfarin, its action may be potentiated by other medications such as anti-hypertensives, antifungals, carbamazepine, steroids, phenytoin, aspirin, and antibiotics such as erythromycin and metronidazole.

If warfarin is being used, a blood sample should be taken to check the INR (International Normalised Ratio - see later chapter on haematology tests). Even if the ratio is higher than it should be, bleeding can usually be stopped with local measures without the need to reverse the warfarin with vitamin K. Only occasionally will reversal be needed. A haematologist should be called if the ratio is very high and bleeding cannot be stopped with local measures. Newer anti-coagulants, rivaroxaban and dabigatran, have no antidote but their effect can be diminished by stopping the medication as they have shorter half-lives.

Once the history has been taken and the patient has bitten on a swab for 15 minutes, the situation can be re-assessed and local anaesthetic with vasoconstrictor can be infiltrated and the wound packed with oxidised surgical gauze and sutures with Vicryl. In persistent cases, a tranexamic acid mouthwash may also be helpful. Also, 500 mg. of tranexamic acid may be given intravenously; this can be very helpful in stopping dental haemorrhage that does not respond to the simplest operative method, but it should be used with caution in the elderly or those with a history of thrombosis.

A patient who has suffered from bleeding should always have a routine full blood count and coagulation screen. Very few patients who present with bleeding will have a platelet or coagulation problem, but a significant number of patients who do have platelet or coagulation problems are initially diagnosed after a dental haemorrhage. These simple screening tests will be automatically reviewed by a haematologist and, if abnormal, will be investigated in more detail.

We have a low threshold for admitting the patient to hospital overnight, particularly if they are elderly, live some distance away or are distressed. Often a small dose of narcotic analgesia (i.e. morphine 5mgs. subcutaneously) will help settle them for the night and help relieve their anxiety.

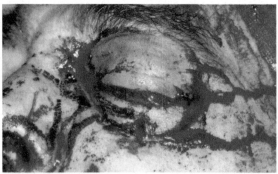

Patient with proptosis, pain opthalmoplegia. There is no sight in the eye.

Bleeding from mouth Key Points

●Patients who are bleeding from sockets must be seen promptly – local anaesthetic with vasoconstrictor, pack with oxidised cellulose gauze, suture sockets, tranexamic acid mouth wash

●If persisted haemorrhage – requires hospital admission

●Identify source of bleeding by sucking out patient's mouth – bite on tightly folded swab

●Obtain full history and medical history

●Drugs contributing to haemorrhage – aspirin, dipyridamole, warfarin

●Warfarin can be potentiated by antihypertensives, antifungals, steroids, antibiotics etc

●Check INR for patient on warfarin – seldom requires Vitamin K for reversal

●New anticoagulants – rivaroxaban and dabigatran have shorter half-life

---

Retrobulbar haemorrhage

An unusual but significant complication of major trauma is a haemorrhage behind the globe of the eye, causing compression on the optic nerve. This may occur after a major traumatic injury, or sometimes because of a more minor impact directly to the eye. You should be aware of this injury as its recognition and prompt management are essential; otherwise, permanent blindness to the affected eye may result.

The signs are proptosis (protrusion of the globe), blindness of the eye, pain and opthalmoplegia (inability to move the eye). The patient should be treated with high-dose steroids and immediate lateral canthotomy and inferior cantholysis to relieve the pressure in the orbit. Should you see these signs, call your specialist

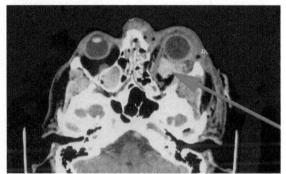

A CT scan shows the collection of blood behind the globe of the eye.

registrar or consultant and advise them of your concern.

When this patient was brought into A&E, no one suspected a retrobulbar haemorrhage or had even examined his eyesight; the main concern was his airway and head injury. The haemorrhage was diagnosed when he was in the CT scanner and subsequent clinical examination confirmed he was blind in the left eye. His orbit was decompressed by lateral canthotomy using local anaesthetic, and he was given high-dose steroids . This was carried out 2½ hours after the injury. He could detect light by the following morning and sight was returned within two days. Much further delay would have meant permanent blindness in that eye.

Early examination and suspicion in peri-orbital trauma can save sight. However, it is uncommon.

13.Examination of the Injured Face

Most patients with suspected facial fractures will present following interpersonal violence. Mostly they will not have any other injuries but may have cuts, abrasions, bruising and swelling. Cuts should be cleaned and sutured; loosened or displaced teeth should be repositioned and splinted. Most patients with fractured mandibles will need admitting to hospital for urgent (but not emergency) surgery.

In the assessment of facial trauma, diagnosis is 80% clinical examination and 20% imaging. Get into the habit of examining the patient before looking at any X-rays or CT scans and don't tell them they have a fracture unless you are absolutely sure. X-rays and CT scans may initially appear to be complicated, but are fairly simple if you approach them methodically (see next chapter). Someone more senior should also examine the patient before any decision is made about the need, or otherwise, for treatment. This may not necessarily be at the same time or visit to the hospital.

Before demonstrating a suggested sequence of examining these patients, it is necessary to consider what we are looking for and what symptoms they might have. We will go through the common fractures in terms of their anatomy, symptoms and signs on clinical examination. Fractures will be considered in the following groups: zygomatic (also called malar) fractures, mandible, dento- alveolar, nasal, and maxillary (also called middle third).

Fractures of the Zygoma (Malar)

The zygomatic fracture is pyramidal shaped and

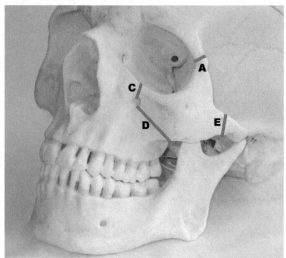

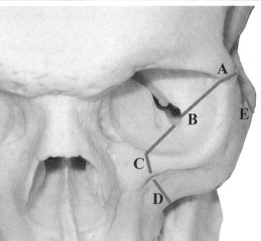

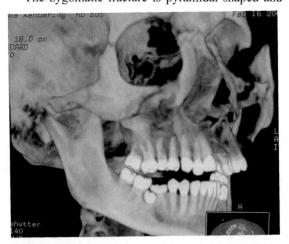

3-D CT scan of mid face fracture. This is almost as bad as it gets. She was a back seat passenger not wearing a seat belt.

involves the zygoma and adjacent bones. Usually, the injury is sustained from a single blow, which is often from a fist. The fracture involves a break at the fronto-zygomatic suture (**A**) which extends through the lateral wall of the orbit and orbital floor (**B**) which is very thin. It then passes though the inferior orbital margin (**C**) to the infra-orbital foramen and then down the zygomatic buttress (**D**) and finally through the zygomatic arch (**E**).

Symptoms

Most patients will have soreness and swelling. Those with severe displacements may have diplopia (double vision). Most will have numbness of the side of the face and difficulty in moving their mandible, particularly laterally.

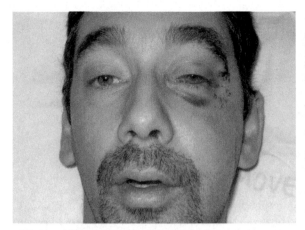

Obvious flattening of left Zygoma

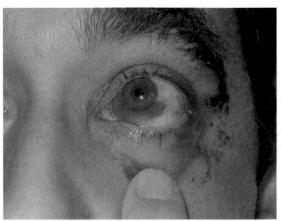

Sub-conjunctival haemorrhage

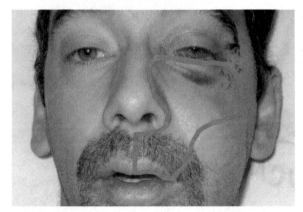

Extent of numbness caused by infra orbital nerve compression

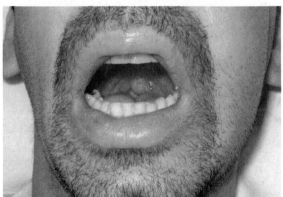

Limitation of opening and lateral jaw movement

Signs to look for

Initially there may be quite severe swelling and bruising, which may be such that assessment may be difficult. Sometimes the eye may be completely closed and it will be necessary to part the eyelids with your fingers to look at it. A crude assessment of vision should be made by asking the patient to count how many fingers you hold up before them. If there is any doubt, they should be referred to an ophthalmic surgeon for assessment and opinion. Many patients will have a sub-conjunctival haemorrhage. This in itself does not indicate a fracture, but it is said that if a posterior limit cannot be seen, there is a higher indication of a fracture.

It is quite possible for there to be quite severe soft tissue swelling without a fracture, and in many cases, it is best to postpone final assessment for a few days until the swelling has mostly subsided. When making this assessment, examine for the following features:-

1. Diplopia. Hold up a fingertip about one metre away and ask the patient to look at it with both eyes and move it throughout the field of vision and ask them to report if they should see double. This may occur if there is disruption of the volume of the orbit in a severe fracture. Diplopia can be measured by an orthoptist in the ophthalmic department using a Hess chart.

2. Cosmetic flattening. This may be obvious, but subtle flattening can best be assessed from above by placing a finger on the malar eminence on both sides and comparing.

3. Step deformity on palpation of the margin of the orbital most easily felt at the inferior orbital margin.

4. Numbness in the distribution of the infra-orbital nerve, i.e. the side of the face and gingivae above the incisors and canine on the affected side. This is because of compression of the nerve in the infra-orbital canal.

5. Decreased opening consequent upon the zygomatic arch pressing on the temporalis muscle and

coronoid process of the mandible.

Management

Usually fractures of the zygoma are elevated using a 'Gillies lift'. An elevator is placed beneath the zygomatic arch through an incision in the temple. Alternatively, a hook can be placed through the cheek. Fixation with a plate increases stability and can be placed at the fronto-zygomatic suture or maxillary buttress fracture. Undisplaced or minimally displaced fractures can be managed conservatively, but elevation and fixation improve the rate of recovery of numbness.

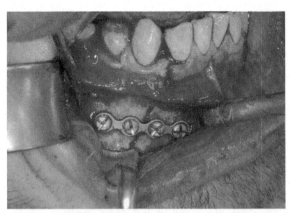

Most mandibular fractures are treated with titanium plates.

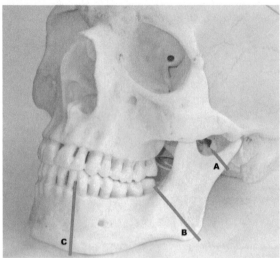

Fractures of the Mandible

The mandible can fracture at any point along its length, but most frequently this occurs:-

A. At the condyle, usually from a blow to the chin from the opposite side. This is the thinnest and, therefore, weakest point of the jaw, and hence most likely to break.

B. At the angle. Here the bone may be thick, but it may be weakened by an unerupted or partly erupted third molar.

C. Parasymphyseal

Symptoms

All patients will complain of pain and discomfort; they may feel their teeth are loose; they will have difficulty chewing and may have difficulty biting their teeth together, opening the mouth or moving the jaw sideways.

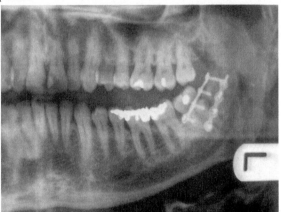

Angle fracture treated with plates - post-op.

Signs to look for

Swelling, bruising, cuts, abrasions and tenderness on palpation over mandible and numbness of the lower lip on the affected side. Intra oral examination may reveal loose teeth, missing teeth, bleeding and splits in the gingivae and above all, derangement of the occlusion; a haematoma in the floor of the mouth suggests a fracture of the mandibular body. Only a dental surgeon will be able to examine the occlusion and make a judgement about whether it is normal for that patient; a consideration of the wear facets on the incisal edges and cusps may need to be made.

Management

Most minimally displaced condylar fractures do not have derangement of the occlusion and can be managed conservatively; the patient can be sent home from A&E and reviewed by the consultant at the clinic. If then there is increasing, rather than improving, pain or occlusal derangement, the jaws can be wired together for two weeks (inter-maxillary fixation) or internally fixed with titanium plates at operation. If the condyles on both sides are fractured, the patient is at risk of developing an anterior open bite. The worse of the two fractures is therefore reduced at operation and fixed with a titanium plate then managed as a unilateral case.

Most other fractures of the mandible are admitted to the ward from A&E for reduction and fixation at a convenient time the next day, but ideally within 24 hours. Most fractures, other than of the condyles, are compound into the mouth and will therefore be given antibiotics.

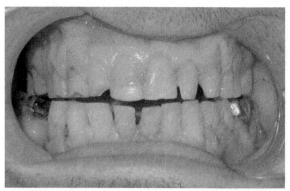

Anterior open bite as a result of bilateral condylar fractures. Obvious only to those with dental training.

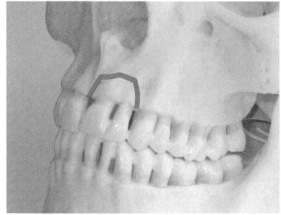

Dento-alveolar fractures

Dento-alveolar fractures are a very common sequelae to falls, sporting accidents and interpersonal violence. They will probably, correctly, be regarded as minor injuries by emergency staff. However, long after broken bones have healed and been forgotten about, a patient may continue to suffer the consequences of lost or damaged teeth. Whereas there are good reasons to delay the treatment of more severe facial fractures, dento-alveolar injuries should be managed immediately to ensure the best results. A common cause for complaints concerns patients with dental injuries who are sent away from an accident and emergency department without being referred to OMFS for urgent assessment and management.

Symptoms

Pain, swelling, bleeding and loose teeth.

Signs to look for

Examine for fractures of the crowns of the teeth, loosening and displacement of the teeth. Look for splits in the attached gingivae. Note which teeth are affected, as this may be necessary for legal reports later. Look for associated lacerations of the soft tissues and pieces

of tooth substance in lip lacerations. If pieces of tooth are missing and the patient may have lost consciousness, a chest X-ray may be necessary to ensure that they have not been inhaled; a low exposure X-ray of overlying soft tissue wounds may show any tooth substance embedded.

Management

Exposed pulps are dressed with dental cement, and loose teeth are repositioned using local anaesthesia. A temporary splint can be made, providing they are not too damaged or the periodontal condition is too bad. The patient is then brought back to the outpatient clinic on the next working day and the teeth more definitively splinted, using orthodontic wires attached with acid etch composite. The patient is then discharged to the care of a primary care or restorative dentist for further follow up, assuming there are no other injuries to be attended to. It is usual for periapical X-rays not to be available out of hours, but the initial urgent treatment is not usually compromised by this.

Fractures of the Nose

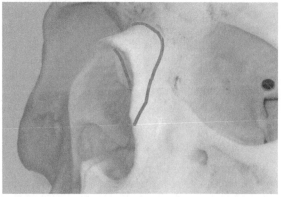

Fractures of the nose are very common and result from interpersonal violence, sporting injuries, and falls. Most isolated nasal fractures may be referred directly

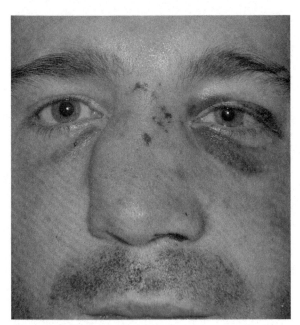

Deviation of dorsum of nose

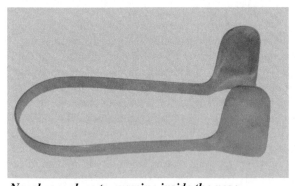

Nasal speculum to examine inside the nose

to the ENT department from the emergency department. We tend to get those which accompany other facial fractures, as a matter of convenience. The nasal bones support the nasal cartilages which support the shape of the external nose, and both may fracture, as may the cartilage of the nasal septum.

Symptoms

Patients with fractures of the nose may complain of pain, swelling, deformity, bleeding or obstruction of the nasal airway.

Signs to look for

The most common complaint will be of nasal deformity. This is best assessed soon after the injury before soft tissue swelling has developed, or several days later when it has subsided. Occasionally, a patient will present who has received a thumping to the nose

on several occasions. In this circumstance, a nasal deformity caused by an old injury can be differentiated from a new one by attempting lateral movement of the nose between gloved fingers and thumb; deformity from an old injury will be firm.

The internal nose should be examined with a good light and a nasal speculum. Nasal obstruction may be caused by a blood clot, a deviation of the nasal septum (ask if they had a clear airway before) or a septal haematoma beneath the perichondrium of cartilaginous septum. Should a haematoma become infected, it can cause necrosis of the cartilage, which may result in loss of support for the dorsum of the nose, and a saddle nose deformity may result. We suggest it would be appropriate to ask an ENT surgeon to see the patient in this circumstance.

A special mention for X-rays. These are contraindicated in nasal fractures. X-rays have a low sensitivity and specificity for identifying nasal fractures. Fractures of the cartilage will not be demonstrated at all, as may many nasal bone fractures. In addition, small vascular markings may appear as fractures to a radiologist and be reported as such when there has been no fracture.

Management

A deviated nose can often be manipulated between fingers and thumb to straighten it without anaesthetic, if done soon after the injury. A septal haematoma beneath the perichondrium of the cartilaginous septum should be drained using local anaesthetic. Otherwise, a deviated nose can be manipulated under general or using local anaesthetic a week later when the swelling has subsided; this will make assessment easier. If the nasal septum remains deviated, causing obstruction to the airway, this is generally managed at a later date by a sub-mucous resection of the septum. This is a routine operation for ENT surgeons.

Fractures of the Maxilla

Maxillary, or middle third (of the face) fractures as they are more accurately described, are nowadays less common than they used to be due to improved car safety. They can be occasionally caused by very severe interpersonal violence.

Maxillary fractures were classified by a Frenchman called René Le Fort at the beginning of the last century. He smashed 35 cadaver faces, dissected them and wrote up his findings. He classified mid face fractures as Le Fort 1,2 or 3. The classification does not have a lot of relevance, as in practice the bones are often smashed into small pieces rather than following the lines of his classification. However, he captured the imagination of surgeons and his classification has been passed from one generation of surgical textbooks to the next, so that most surgeons have heard of it but few will understand it.

The Le Fort 2 level fracture is the least uncommon. A Le Fort 1 fracture requires a very concentrated force at a low level of the mid-face, which is unusual. A Le Fort 3 is caused by a severe force and involves separating most of the facial bones from the cranial base. Anyone sustaining this degree of trauma may be suffered a significant head injury. This may not be noticed initially and the effect may be subtle, such as poor concentration, lethargy or depressed mood.

Symptoms

The patients will probably, but not necessarily, have severe facial swelling and bruising. Their eyes may be completed closed with oedema, they will have been bleeding from the nose and the mouth and they will have a disturbed occlusion and loose teeth. Many of these injuries will have been caused by severe trauma, which may have also caused other injuries. The patient might have a neck injury, so a cervical collar will have been placed to stabilise the neck. This should only be removed after the neck has been X rayed and examined by an orthopaedic surgeon. The airway may be at risk, so the patient may have been intubated. Usually, the facial injuries themselves will not be life threatening, so other injuries will take priority.

Signs to look for

Examination may be difficult if the patient is intubated and wearing a cervical collar. If not intubated, examine the dentition and occlusion, examine for numbness and look at the eyes to check vision is OK. The diagnosis of maxillary fracture is easily made by holding the anterior maxilla with a gloved hand and attempting a differential movement of the maxilla while holding the bridge of the nose between the finger and thumb of the other hand.

Management

Definitive surgery for a maxillary fracture may be delayed for a couple of weeks while the swelling subsides and other injuries, such as orthopaedic and head injuries, are dealt with.
Occasionally, bleeding from the maxilla will be difficult to control, in which case you will need to call someone senior. Patients with head injuries will probably need a CT scan, and the most useful thing you can do is ask them to include the face in the initial scan. Coronal views showing the orbital floor and volume

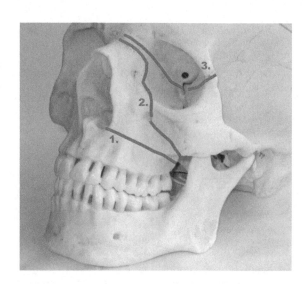

Le Fort Classification: 1. Low level, separates the dento-alveolar segment from the rest of the maxilla, is very unusual as it requires a severe force in a very concentrated area of the lower part of maxilla above the teeth. 2. The most common. It is a pyramidal fracture across nasal bones, through orbits and across buttress of the zygoma. 3. Separation of whole of face from cranial base, a very severe injury; many with this may not survive the head injury. The pattern may be different on each side, there may be fractures at several levels on the same side, and the bones may be comminuted into small pieces.

will be most useful.

Although definitive surgery may be delayed, it may be necessary to take them to theatre that day to do a tracheotomy to secure the airway. Loose teeth can then be removed, severely displaced fractures can be temporarily approximated with wires, and lacerations sutured.

Definitive surgery may vary from as little as a couple of plates placed within the mouth for a patient with an intact dental arch and little displacement of the occlusion, to major surgery involving open reduction of the fractures from both intra and extra oral approaches.

Now that we have briefly described the main facial fractures that you will come across, you should have a rough idea of what you are looking for. We will now go through a sequence of the steps you should go through when you see a patient with facial trauma.

Examination of the face

1. Examine soft tissues

Draw a rough diagram of lacerations, abrasions and other skin marks and include measurements.

2. Examine the eyes

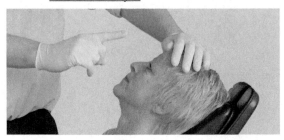

Look for sub-conjunctival haemorrhage (redness below the conjunctiva), and level of the pupil compared with the opposite side. Steady the patient's head and ask them to follow your finger, held one metre away, through all movements to check ocular movements (particularly upwards) and ask if they have any double vision.

A malar fracture may cause sub-conjunctival bleeding; a severe fracture may cause a lowering of the orbital floor and hence the globe of the eye. A large change in orbital volume in such an injury can lead to diplopia and may entrap orbital contents (particularly inferior rectus muscle) in the fractured floor, causing limitation of upward gaze.

3. Palpate the orbital margins

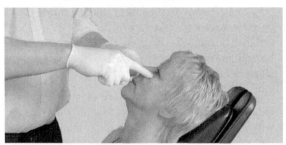

Palpate the orbital rims for evidence of a step deformity which would be felt if there were a fracture of the Zygoma or much less commonly a Le Fort 2 of the maxilla.

Before examining the face

Take a history

 Record the time you saw them

Can they remember the incident?
How did the injury occur?
Time of injury
Anyone else hurt?
Wearing seat belt?
Alcohol involved?
Past medical history
Social history

 Direct questions

 Headache

Any loss of consciousness?
Nausea or vomiting?
Vision OK? Diplopia
Numbness of face
Police involvement

 Also examine & record

 Injuries elsewhere

Glasgow coma scale
(in practice this will already have been done by casualty doctor before you were called.)

4. Look for flattening of the Zygoma

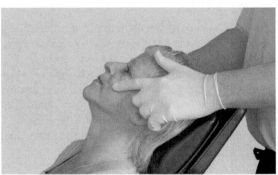

This is best achieved by standing behind the patient and looking and palpating the prominence of the cheek and comparing the two sides. Flattening is best assessed either very soon after the injury, before swelling has started, or several days later when it has started to subside.

5. Check nose

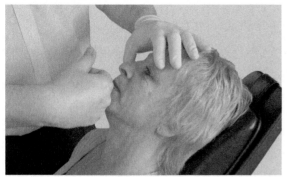

Is the nose deviated and if so does this predate the injury or is it new? Check the nasal airway by obstructing each nostril in turn and feeling for the breath with your finger.

6. Examine inside the nose

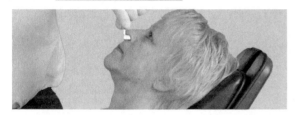

Use a nasal speculum to look for a septal swelling which may be a haematoma needing draining. Don't bother if there is no obvious nasal injury.

7. Examine for numbness

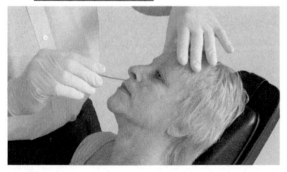

Check for numbness in the distribution of the infra orbital nerve on the face which usually accompanies a malar or maxillary fracture. Remember not to miss the gingivae above the incisor and canine teeth which will be involved. The mental nerve may have been injured in fractures of the mandible.

8. Is the maxilla firm ?

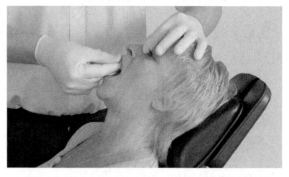

Wearing gloves, hold the nasal bridge and anterior maxillary alveolus firmly and try to elicit a differential movement

9. Examine the mouth

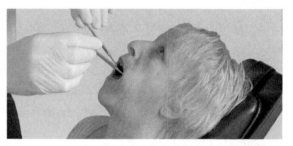

Look for loose and broken teeth, derangement of the occlusion, tears in the soft tissues and particularly of the gingivae. Using gloved hands, try to elicit movement across any part of the mandible you suspect may be fractured but are not sure. Check for mouth opening and lateral movement. Feel for tenderness of the temporomandibular joint.

29.6.13 00.15 Hr.

Robert Andrews 20♂

- alleged assault at approx 10.00 pm.

2 blows to left side of face

- not been drinking can remember incident

LOC°   nausea°   vomiting°

only facial injury

o/e alert & orientated GCS=15

° SC haemorrhage, normal eye movement

° diplopia   ° malar flattening

Nasal airway patient

maxilla firm

° facial numbness

left lip swollen, 2 cm laceration through skin & vermillion of lip - not throu to mouth

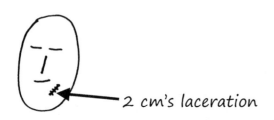

— 2 cm's laceration

IOE

Mobility between 12

1 # enamel just into dentine

Premature occlusion L buccal segment

° floor mouth haematoma

OPG

Confirms # R parasymphysis

Between 1 & 2

Plan

Inform specialist registrar on call

1.   Suture laceration LA

1.   Admit to ward

1.   IV fluid

1.   Nil by mouth for theatre am

Treat

LA lidocaine/adrenaline

1 X 2.0 mls cartridge

2 cm laceration closed with deep 3/0 Vicryl & 5/0 ethilon to skin

R Undergreen.

ROB UNDERGREEN

OMFS CT2

14. Imaging for Facial Fractures

Most patients with fractures of the facial skeleton will have the fracture diagnosed from the history and symptoms confirmed by clinical examination. In practically all cases, an X-ray examination will be made to confirm the diagnosis and to aid in the planning of surgery. For fractures of the mandible, the orthopantomograph (OPG) will combine the most radiological information with best radiological hygiene. In most cases, the OPG alone will suffice, but some fractures of the angle or condyle will not be visualised and a posterior-anterior (PA) image will be used as well. Although most cases will be obvious from clinical examination, many surgeons will feel more comfortable having two images at right angles.

You will already know the OPG is a tomogram. The principle is that the X-ray source and sensor rotate around the subject so that radiopaque structures (cervical spine in this case) not of interest are outside the focal trough. This decreases interference with the image of the area being examined. The main limitation of the OPG for trauma patients is that the patient must be able to stand or sit in the machine, so it may not be suitable for those with severe or multiple injuries, especially if they are wearing a cervical collar because of a neck injury. For the PA view of the mandible, the X-ray sensor or film plate is placed in front of the face and the rays pass from behind the patient forward at 90° to the sensor. CT scans may often be used for displaced condylar fractures.

The other common facial fracture is of the malar (zygoma). CT scans are usually used by most surgeons for all mid-face fractures, but you may well find that many feel comfortable managing simple malar fractures with just a plain X-ray. The image used will be the 15° occipito-mental (OM). Here the principle is that X-rays will pass through the occiput to the sensor, which is at 15° to the perpendicular of the film. The patient is positioned with his chin and nose touching the sensor. This should produce a clear image of the bony margins of the mid-face. The patient must be able to stand, sit, or lie face down. An image made with the patient lying on his back and the film behind the head will give an indistinct view of the mid-face.

In most cases where you are asked to see a patient with facial trauma, images will have already have been obtained. If not, an OPG and 15° OM are all you need to request. In many hospitals now, a CT scan will be used for most fractures. Remember, it is always good

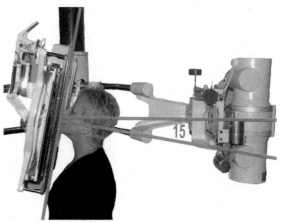

Making 15° OM image

practice to get into the habit of examining the patient and making a clinical diagnosis before looking at images.

Computerised Tomography (CT) is an X-ray image made using the tomography principle. The X-ray source and sensors are located in a ring, which spirals around the patient as they move through on a platform. In older scanners, the image is acquired in an axial plain, and coronal and sagittal scans are reconstructed by the computer. With modern scans, a 3D data set is used and the image can be viewed in three dimensions. This gives the surgeon a more realistic image of what will be encountered at operation. This is of particular value in fractures around the orbit.

Do not miss the opportunity to see CT scans being made; the best way to see the images is on the video screen in the scanner centre with the radiologist or the radiographer showing you. The traditional technique of printing images onto film is now obsolete as digital imaging systems are built into hospitals using video screens to view images.

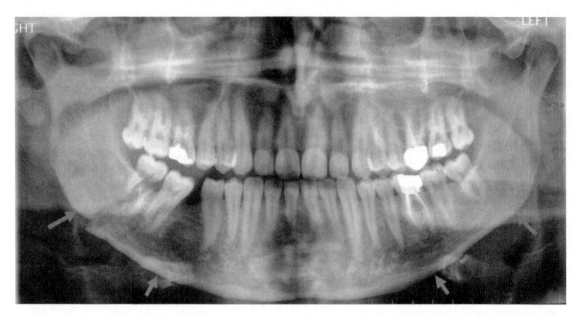

Always check the name of the patient on the film, the date and orientation. Examine all the margins of the mandible sequentially, the most common sites of fracture being the condylar neck, angle and parasymphysis. Check that your diagnosis fits with the clinical findings. The fracture here is obvious at the right angle involving the second molar tooth. The fracture is often seen as a double lucency which represents the break through the buccal and lingual cortex of the mandible, and not two separate fractures.

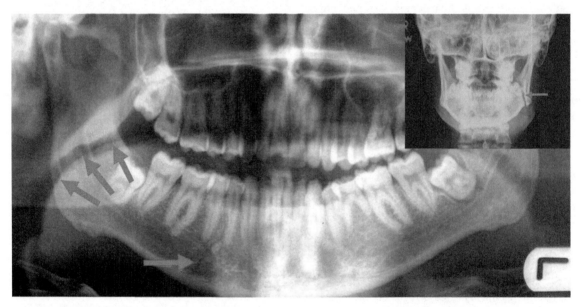

OPG Potential Problems: *To the untutored observer who has not properly examined the patient the pharyngeal air shadow can sometimes be suspected as a fracture. This is marked at the right angle, however you can see that it extends beyond the mandible. The fracture marked at the right body is clear but can you see a fracture at the left angle? No, neither can we. However, a PA view (X rays passing from posterior to anterior) clearly shows the fracture. Sometimes an angle fracture will not show clearly. However, this will be suspected from clinical examination and the taking of a PA film as a routine is not justified. The OPG does not image the symphysis well because of the superimposition of the cervical spine. This can be imaged with an intra-oral occlusal film.*

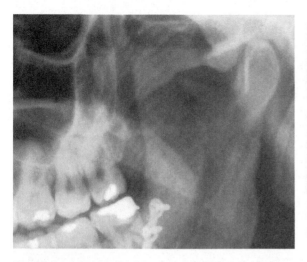

Detail from an OPG shows the condylar fracture but ...

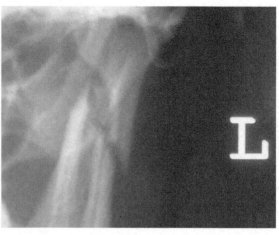

... it is more clearly seen on the detail from the PA film.

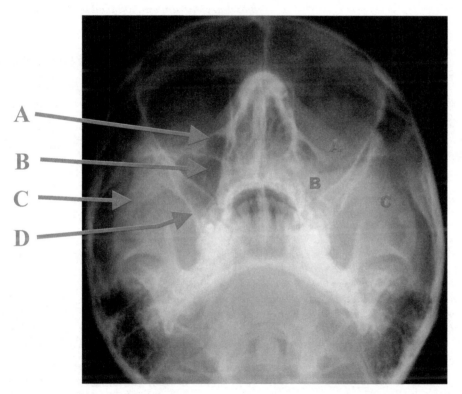

15° Occipital-mental of patient with fracture of left malar. Compare the injured with the uninjured side, looking at: A. The rim of the orbit for loss of continuity. B. The maxillary antrum for a fluid level or opacity caused by blood. . C. The zygomatic arch D. The lateral maxillary wall for loss of continuity. You can see that on the left side there is severe disruption of the orbital rim, loss of opacity of the antrum, a break in the zygomatic arch, and it is difficult to make out the lateral antral wall clearly. A widening of the fronto-zygomatic suture is also frequently seen in zygomatic fractures. However, the suture can often be quite prominent anyway if the x-rays are angled with the film so as to accentuate it.

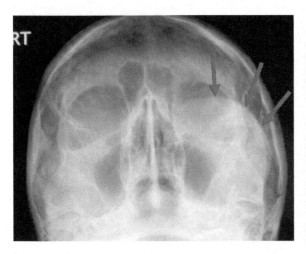

15° OM potential problems. The maxillary antrum may appear opaque from severe facial swelling or haematoma in the soft tissues. Look for soft tissue shadow as marked above.

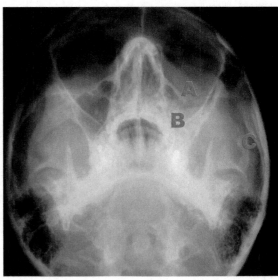

15° OM. A. Buckled orbital rim B. Opaque maxillary antrum due to blood and displaced bone from lateral antral wall C. Fracture of zygomatic arch

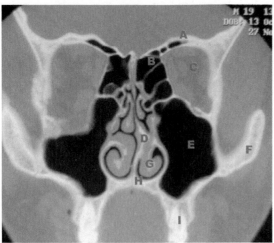

Coronal CT of mid face. A. Cranial base B. Ethmoidal air cells C. Orbit (behind the globe of the eye), the medial, lateral, superior and inferior rectus muscles and the optic nerve may be seen as slight opacities D. Nasal septum (deviated) E. Maxillary antrum F. Prominence of Zygoma G. Inferior concha H. Bony palate I. Molar tooth

The scan shows an isolated fracture of the right orbital floor (orbital blow out) with part of the orbital contents bulging into the maxillary antrum.

Let us compare the quality and clarity of the 15° occipito-mental plain x-ray 3-D images, axial CT slice and 3-D CT image of a patient who has suffered a fractured malar (zygoma).

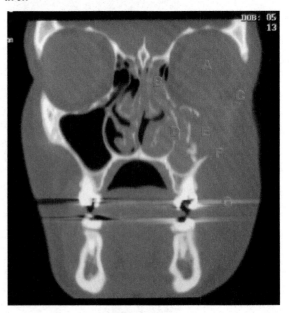

Coronal CT scan same patient. A. Globe of the eye in the same position as uninjured side B. Ethmoids filled with opaque blood, inferior orbital wall fractured C. Prominence of Zygoma missing from same plane as uninjured side D. Blood in the nose and lateral nasal wall fractured E. Bone and blood in the antrum F Lateral antral wall missing G. Artefacts from amalgam fillings

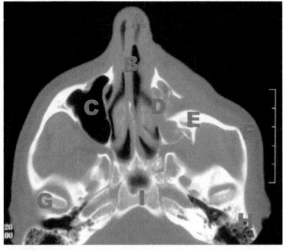

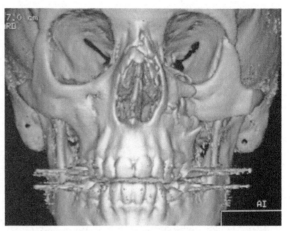

The computer can be used to adjust the view of the 3-D image. Note the artefacts caused by amalgam fillings.

Axial CT scan of the same patient. A. External nose B. Nasal septum C. Maxillary antrum on uninjured side D. Position of antrum on injured side showing opaque blood and bone fragments within E. Prominence of Zygoma displaced inwards F. Zygomatic arch G. Condyles of mandible H. Mastoid air cells I. Cervical spine

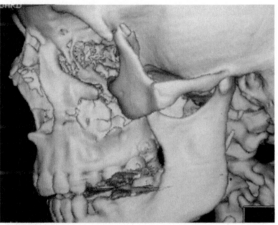

3-D image reconstructed from the CT scans of the same patient with fracture of the left malar.

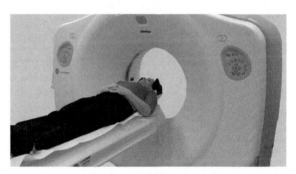

Patient in CT scanner

15. <u>Wound Closure - Skin Suturing</u>

Some of your most satisfying work will be attending to soft tissue lacerations. The best time to close facial lacerations is immediately, using local analgesia, although severe, multiple and complex soft tissue injuries may need a general anaesthetic for the best cosmetic result.

Children require special consideration, rather than any special skill. In most cases, the injuries will result from falls or dog bites. A small child is usually best admitted to the children's ward, the paediatrician informed, and arrangements made for a paediatric anaesthetist to administer the following morning. This should preferably be the first case on an emergency operating list so that the child is not starved for a long period. With some small wounds, it will be acceptable for a dressing to be put in place and for the child to go home with the parents and return first thing in the morning.

For children, we always obtain consent for "examination under anaesthesia, clean and repair wounds as necessary". It is much better not to distress the child and parents with a detailed and uncomfortable deep examination of a wound or intra oral examination. All will be revealed more easily later under general anaesthesia. You may resist the temptation to place absorbable sutures through the epidermis of the skin rather than nylon, which, although it needs to be removed, gives a much better cosmetic result. Sometimes an uncooperative child may need a second anaesthetic five days later for removal of nylon sutures. This will usually be better than compromising a good aesthetic result by placing absorbable sutures, which may leave point scars on the skin. We never use fibrin glue to close wounds on children, as the result is usually inferior to nylon sutures or synthetic monofilament resorbable sutures, such as Monocryl.

As with all practical tasks, acclimatise yourself to the instruments and materials before you first approach a patient, and get the feel of them by practising suturing on a manikin. We preferentially use pig skin for this purpose as it allows the dermis and epidermis to be closed separately. The layers are not so easily defined as in human skin, which is therefore easier to sew.

You should initially examine the patient, ensure that there are no other facial or dental injuries, and record the injuries in the notes. If the wound is deep

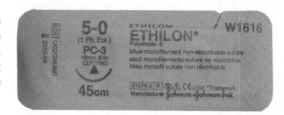

Polyamide (Nylon) trade name Ethilon. This is monofilament, i.e. it is not braided and therefore cleaner and excites very little local inflammation. It is therefore suitable for a good cosmetic result on the face but needs to be removed in 5 to 7 days. It is strong but brittle and can easily break when it is being tied. The material retains a memory so the knots can easily come undone so you need to pace 2 throws in both directions. Use 5-0 (which is very fine) for most areas of the face where a good cosmetic result is needed, and use 4-0 elsewhere such as the neck.

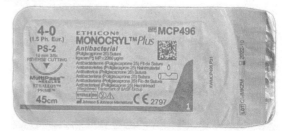

Monocryl is synthetic and resorbable. Use for skin where you don't want to have to remove the sutures.

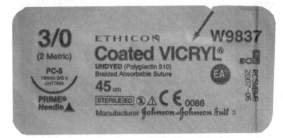

Untreated Polyglactin (Vicryl) is stronger, dissolves more slowly and is easier to handle as it is less fragile and likely to break. We would use it where we want the wound to be stronger and watertight as for orthognathic or cancer surgery or just for strength as when putting deep sutures in the scalp. It is coated with a copolymer of lactide and glycolide which slows loss of tensile strength and promotes more rapid absorption when the strength is lost. It is also coated with calcium stearate, which helps with tissue passage and smoothness of the knot tie.

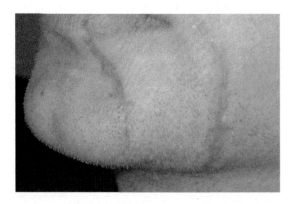

Dirt tattoo caused by inadequate wound cleaning before suturing

5/0 or 4/0 polypropylene such as Prolene or nylon such as Ethilon. The main mistake made by new surgeons is to place too many sutures; every suture is a foreign body which can promote infection, and deep absorbable sutures can lead to stitch abscesses. Always use just the minimum needed to oppose the skin edges neatly.

Usually, patients with facial lacerations should not be given antibiotics. This policy may be varied if the patient has deep contaminated wounds or other

or penetrating underlying structures such as the facial nerve, parotid duct or alar nasal cartilages may be involved; in these cases you should get help from your superiors.

Where tissue is missing, it may be better to allow that part to heal by secondary intention rather than stretch the skin, which may cause unsightly contractions later. This is particularly so around the eye; tension of skin may lead to ectropion (distortion of the lower eyelid pulled away from the conjunctiva), which is unsightly. For sewing wounds of the eyelid, consult with an oculoplastic surgeon, if one is available.

Reassure the patient and make sure your assistant has the correct instruments ready. Ensure the patient is in a comfortable position, that there are adequate surgical drapes in place and that you have a good operating light. You should then apply local anaesthetic. We use lignocaine and adrenaline from dental cartridges because the dental needles are so fine. The wound should be thoroughly cleaned with surgical swabs and sterile saline, ensuring any road dirt is scrubbed from the wounds and any grazed skin; otherwise, it may produce unsightly skin tattooing. Any blood clot should be removed; the wound edges should be rubbed clean until fresh bleeding occurs.

The wound should then be closed with sutures. If it is deep, any dead space should be closed with 4/0 treated polyglactin, such as Vicryl Rapide or a similar material, using the minimum number of sutures. Following this, the dermis should be closed using the same material with the knots buried away from the surface. Finally, the epidermis should be closed with

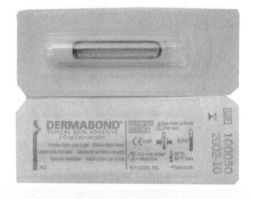

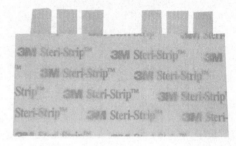

Cyanoacrylate glue (Dermobond) and adhesive tape (Steri-Strip) can be used as a temporary measure or as a definitive closure for a previously battle scarred uncooperative drunk. Tape can be used for very superficial cuts or to augment the strength of a sutured wound. Resist the temptation to use either as a definitive treatment for a small, tired and fractious child who is uncooperative. The glue will give a less than ideal tissue closure with a sub optimal cosmetic result and the child will have the strips off before they get to the bus stop. Get them back the next day and suture properly with a GA, even if it means a second anaesthetic for suture removal. Mother will want the very best result.

associated compound bony injury. The A&E nurse will normally check the patient's tetanus immunisation status and give a booster if required. Facial skin wounds are usually better without dressings, especially adherent ones. Chloramphenicol cream applied to the wound twice daily by the patient may help reduce secondary infection and prevent scab formation; this will make suture removal easier.

Arrangements should be made with the patient for the sutures to be removed in about 5 days. This can be by the GP's nurse or in the outpatient department, depending upon convenience, the patient's wishes and local policy. The patients should be advised that non-absorbable sutures are used on the surface of the skin as they produce a better cosmetic result than dissolvable ones. However, if you are suturing the scalp within the hairline, this will not matter.

How to describe a suture

A: *The USP (United States Pharmacopeia) size definition of the thread diameter. You will only use 3/0 (0.2mm diam.) 4-0 (.015 mm diam.) or 5-0 (0.1 mm diam). The larger the number the finer the thread. Use 4-0 for deep sutures in the face unless the wound is on the scalp, in which case you will need something much stronger.* **B**: *The manufacturer.* **C**: *The trade name for the suture.* **D**: *The number for the individual suture.* **E**: *The parent company* **F**: *The material the suture is made of, its filament type and whether it is absorbable.* **G**: *The length of the thread.* **H**: *Diagram of the needle shape, laterally and in cross section. Needles may be straight or curved, cutting or round bodied. You will use exclusively curved cutting needles* **I**: *Description of the needle in words*

Polyglactin braided absorbable suture material (Vicryl) is the most commonly used in our department. There is Vicryl Rapide which means that it is Vicryl which has been treated with gamma rays to increase the speed of absorption. It dissolves fairly quickly but gives only minimal support and is ideal for dento-alveolar surgery, where soft tissue flap support is needed for only a few days. It is also used for deep sutures beneath the skin surface, which likewise need only minimal support and quick absorption is an advantage. It is only fair in handling quality, being fairly brittle; it will easily break if you pull too tightly when tying. However, it knots fairly well; the knots are stable and don't loosen.

So if you want this suture (which you frequently will) you would ask the nurse for a '3/0 Vicryl Rapide on a curved cutting needle please.' Alternately, if you can remember it, you can just ask for the suture number: 'a W9919 please.'

How to place a skin suture

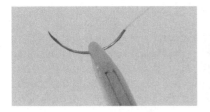

1. Hold the suture needle in the centre at 90 degrees. Try not to deviate from this position; you will find it difficult at first but in time this practice will pay off.

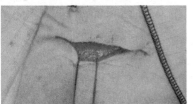

2. Before closing a traumatic wound ensure that it is clean by washing with surgical swabs soaked in saline. Close any deep tissue space with minimal deep sutures. Avoid causing unnecessary trauma to the skin with the forceps.

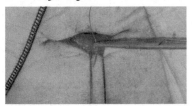

3. First place a suture through the dermis from below upwards; the aim is to bury the knot away from the skin surface. Hold the skin margin closest to you and pass a Vicryl suture needle towards you through the dermal layer.

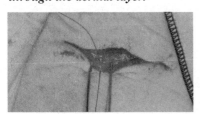

4. and pull the suture through towards you.

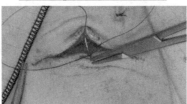

5. Now do the opposite. Pass the needle through the dermis furthest away from you, from above down and pull it through towards you.

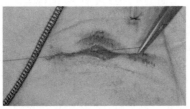

6. Tie the knot 2 throws one way & one the other. The knot should be buried with the knotted strands both the same side of the superficial strand of the loop.

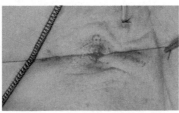

7' Tighten the knot and cut it short.

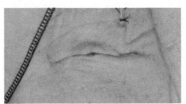

8. Place more sutures to close the rest of the dermis. Use minimal sutures; beginners usually place too many.

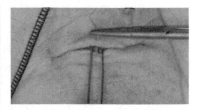

9. Pass a nylon suture through the epidermal layer furthest away from you from above down.

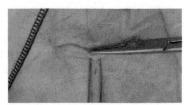

10. Then through the epidermis closest to you from below up.

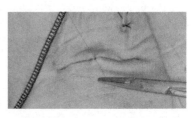

11. Tie the knot two throws one way, one the other and another two the first way as this material is inclined to slip and the suture needs an extra throw to secure it.

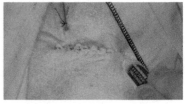

12. Apply chloramphenicol cream and give the patient a supply to take home to apply twice daily. Superficial sutures should be removed in 5 to 7 days on the face.

16. Medical Emergencies

A medical emergency is a sudden or unexpected event which is potentially life threatening. You will be required to undertake continuing training in these subjects during your time in the hospital.

You are most likely to have to deal with a medical emergency in the outpatient clinic, possibly when you are carrying out minor surgery using local anaesthetic. Although the chance of this happening is low, it is still higher than when working in dental practice. Many patients will be referred to the hospital for minor surgery because of co-existing medical problems. That the situations to be described are unusual makes it even more important that you should be up to date with the procedures necessary to recognise and deal with them. You should also know how adverse events might be minimised.

You should be familiar with the recommendations of the Resuscitation Council who provide guidance on their website on the practice and training for cardiopulmonary resuscitation in primary dental care. These guidelines are reviewed regularly and updated according to available evidence; they should be your bible for resuscitation throughout your career and should be memorised for postgraduate examinations as well as for practice.

However, these recommendations are for a dental surgery and assume no familiarity with gaining intravenous access. In the hospital, IV access will be second nature and there should be a 'medical emergency team' who can be called in all cases where a patient is in danger. They have replaced the concept of the 'cardiac arrest' team, who were called when a patient arrested. The medical emergency team is there to act before the patient is in extremis and prevent cardiac arrest, as well as managing it wherever possible.

All the equipment needed for dealing with these emergencies should be in the resuscitation trolley. There should be one available in each clinical area, including the wards and outpatient departments. This will include drugs, airways and IV access equipment.

Vaso-vagal syncope

Vaso-vagal syncope is unlikely to be life threatening, but it has to be considered here because it is the most common cause of loss of consciousness in the surgery. The diagnosis is easy because it is usually preceded by characteristic prodromal symptoms of light-headedness, feeling hot, sweating and restlessness, often involving rubbing of the face. Recovery is rapid once the patient is tipped back in the chair so that their legs are higher than their head; this can be accelerated by lifting their legs up. We find that loss of consciousness is usually prevented by tipping the patient in response to the prodromal signs. If the patient actually loses consciousness because the prodromal signs have been missed, they may start convulsing; this quickly ceases when consciousness recovers and should not be considered as an epileptic seizure.

The process occurs as a result of vagus activity causing a slowing of the heart accompanied by vasodilation producing a decrease in cerebral blood flow. This is most likely to occur when minor oral surgery is performed on a patient who has not eaten for some time and is very apprehensive about the surgery. The reaction is likely to be triggered by pain, prolonged operating time, and the negative emotion of loss of confidence in the surgeon's ability to achieve adequate analgesia. An apprehensive patient may react to the tactile pressure of exodontia as if in pain, even if optimal anaesthesia has been obtained; this may be exacerbated by repeatedly poking the area and asking if they can feel it. An inexperienced or bad nurse assistant can almost talk a patient into passing out by repeatedly asking after their welfare during the operation.

Recovery can be helped by providing oxygen through a face mask. Once consciousness is regained, treatment can then be finished with the patient in a slightly reclined or horizontal position.

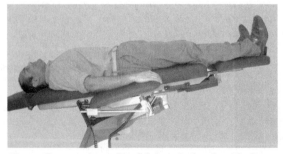

Your first action should be to tip the chair or operating table down so that the patient's legs are raised.

Other relatively benign causes of loss of consciousness are postural hypotension and hyperventilation. Postural hypotension usually occurs as a result of standing up rapidly, usually pre-disposed to by anti-hypertensive medication. Hyperventilation resulting from anxiety can cause light-headedness but rarely loss of consciousness.

Anaphylaxis

Anaphylaxis is a severe allergic reaction resulting in IgE mediated de-granulation of mast cells with the release of histamine. The histamine causes vasodilatation of arterioles and bronchospasm, leading to a decrease in blood pressure and respiratory distress. Decrease in blood pressure may lead to collapse and cardiac arrest. The bronchospasm may proceed to respiratory arrest and be followed by cardiac arrest.

Anaphylaxis may result from allergy to a medication or its additives. It may result from systemic or topical administration or even to latex gloves.

The patient may (or may not) have a flushed appearance, urticaria, angioedema, vomiting, wheezing, stridor, hoarse voice or loss of consciousness. The reaction may vary from mild, producing little more than a flushed appearance, to cardiopulmonary arrest and death.

In severe cases, the patient should be reclined, given oxygen at 15 L/min. and 0.5 ml. of 1:1000 adrenaline intramuscularly into the antero-lateral thigh. The medical emergency team should be called. The adrenaline may be repeated after five minutes if blood pressure or adequate respiration are not maintained. An intravenous line should be put in quickly, and Hartmann's solution or 0.9% saline given to restore blood pressure. Antihistamines and steroids may be given initially in milder cases or after resuscitation in

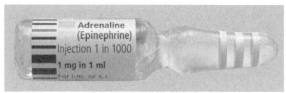

Adrenaline. 1:1000 for anaphylaxis

more severe cases. Immediate resuscitation, according to the ABCDE approach (see next chapter) will be needed if there is a loss of consciousness or breathing stops.

Asthma and COPD

You will have to see many patients who have asthma or chronic obstructive pulmonary disease (COPD). Most patients will be very knowledgeable about the pattern and severity of their disease. In the unlikely circumstance that a patient suffers an acute exacerbation of their asthma in the clinic or during minor surgery, they will usually respond to salbutamol, delivered through their own inhaler. If they are very short of breath, they may not be able to inhale an adequate dose from an inhaler alone; in this case, it may be necessary to use a spacer to deliver the salbutamol.

Severe asthma is indicated by the patient being unable to speak a sentence in one breath, or having a respiratory rate increased to 25 per minute or more, or a tachycardia of over 110 per minute. Then they will need salbutamol and oxygen through a nebuliser. By this stage, you should have called the medical emergency team.

You will occasionally see patients with COPD, which is so severe that they use regular home nebulisers or oxygen. Their minor surgery or dental

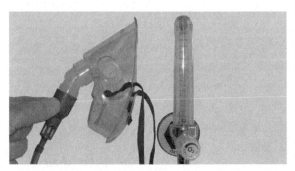

Oxygen should be available on the wall of all the surgeries you use.

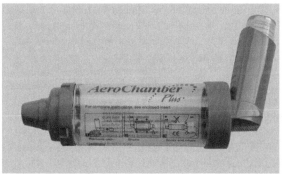

Salbutamol inhaler attached to a spacer which improves the efficiency of drug delivery to the airways.

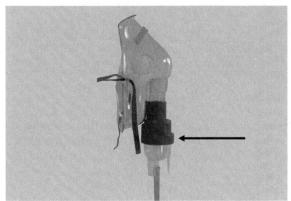

Salbutamol, placed in a nebuliser (arrow) attached to a standard face mask and air supply, is the most efficient way to dilate the airways in severe asthma.

extractions are best done under local anaesthetic in the operating theatre, under the supervision of an anaesthetist with oxygen administered with nasal cannulae, heart monitoring, an IV line and possibly some light sedation.

Epilepsy

You would normally be aware of a patient with epilepsy from taking their previous medical history. Most are very well controlled, but you should still know what to do if a patient should have a grand-mal seizure. This should be fairly easy to recognise. Before becoming unconscious, the patient may have a brief 'aura' which is followed by rigidity and possibly cyanosis. After that, there will be jerking movements of the limbs and possible urinary incontinence. The attack may last for a few minutes and be followed by floppiness. Eventually, they become conscious again, but possibly confused.

The patient should be given oxygen at 15 L/min. while fitting, and attempts should be made to avoid them injuring themselves. However, they should not be physically restrained and nothing should be put into their mouth, not even an oral airway. If fitting continues for longer than five minutes, buccal midazolam should be administered and IV access established.
Hospital admission will be needed if the patient needs such medication to control the fit; they should be reviewed by the medical team. If the fitting continues, the medical emergency team should be called. They would normally give IV lorazepam as the next line in management. Occasionally a fit may be triggered by hypoglycaemia so the blood sugar should be checked and if below 3 mmols./ L glucose or glucagon should

be given.

Should a patient remain unresponsive after the fit and have no sign of breathing or pulse, cardio-pulmonary resuscitation should be started according to the ABCDE principle (described in the next chapter).

Hypoglycaemia

Diabetic patients will normally be able to recognise the symptoms of hypoglycaemia. They will feel a general uneasiness and malaise with fatigue and nervousness. This can normally be reversed quickly by taking a drink containing glucose; milk with three teaspoons of sugar added will be very suitable or a sweet (not low calorie) drink or snack. If the symptoms are not recognised, it may progress to trembling, headache, tachycardia, aggression, confusion, convulsions and coma. A blood glucose estimation will confirm a level of below 3 mmols. per litre. However, as soon as these signs are seen in a diabetic patient, they should be given a glucose drink if they can swallow.

If the patient should become unconscious, they should be given either glucagon, 1 mg. intramuscularly, or 50 ml. of intravenous glucose, through a large bore needle. Glucagon is preferable, as the glucose solution is highly irritant if any of it is inadvertently injected outside of the vein. This will be needed rarely, as most cases will respond to a glucose drink and the emergency team will not be needed.

Acute Coronary Syndromes

Many patients will be referred to hospital for routine dental extraction simply because they have a history of ischaemic heart disease. A patient with angina will probably carry their own glyceryl trinitrate

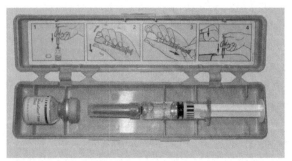

Glucagon pre-loaded in syringe for emergency injection

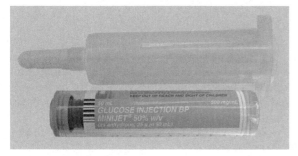

Glucose injection

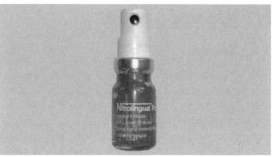

Glyceryl Trinitrate

(GTN) sublingual spray. Should they feel any chest pain, they may well be able to use it to get relief. If this is not unusual for them, they can continue with their treatment. Where the pain is prolonged, the patient should be given oxygen through a face mask and transferred to the Accident and Emergency department or Medical Admissions Unit for an ECG and assessment by a physician.

Patients who have stable angina or a history of a previous myocardial infarct may be treated under local anaesthetic satisfactorily in the outpatient facility. However, where there is unstable angina, a history of a very recent infarction or severe heart failure, treatment should be carried out in the operating theatre using local anaesthetic An anaesthetist can then supervise their cardiac status with an ECG and give oxygen with a nasal cannula. Remember that a diabetic or someone elderly may experience only limited pain with a myocardial infarction, or even none; your threshold for referral for a medical opinion must be low. In every case of chest pain, monitor their pulse and respiratory rate. A pulse rate over 100 should be regarded with suspicion, and a respiratory rate of over 15 per minute should start your alarm bells.

Myocardial Infarction is a diagnosis made by ECG and cardiac enzyme (Troponin T) estimation. Clinically, however, the pain will be like angina but more severe, more crushing and more prolonged. The pain will occur in the centre of the chest and radiate across to the shoulders and down the arms. The patient may become short of breath, cold and clammy, nauseous and have a weak pulse and blood pressure may fall.

The medical emergency team should be called immediately and GTN should be given, followed by 300 mg. aspirin crushed or chewed. Oxygen should be given at 15L/min and if consciousness is lost, resuscitation as the ABCDE approach should be started.

17. <u>Resuscitation</u>

Introduction

Cardiopulmonary resuscitation (CPR) comprises those procedures used to revive heart and lung function where they have ceased. Cardiopulmonary collapse has many causes, but in most cases it will follow acute heart failure because of myocardial infarction ('heart attack'). There are situations where resuscitation would not be appropriate, such as when death is expected in someone very ill. Here the attempt would be pointless and cruel; the patient may have previously indicated that they do not wish to be resuscitated. For inpatients who fall into this category, a Do Not Attempt Resuscitation (DNAR) form will have been completed; this is very unlikely for OMFS patients.

Myocardial infarction (MI) is caused by occlusive thrombus at the site of rupture or erosion of a plaque of atheroma in one of the coronary arteries. The process may take several hours and may be salvaged with clot dissolving drugs if they are administered early. Many patients will have the classic symptoms: crushing

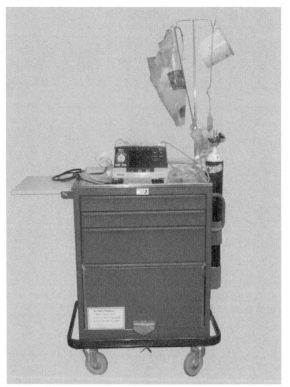

Resuscitation trolley. You can see an oxygen cylinder, intravenous fluids, a defibrillator and a sharps disposal bin.

central chest pain radiating down the (usually) left arm, shortness of breath and collapse. However, it is possible to have a painless infarction, particularly in diabetics and the elderly; the patient may initially have just shortness of breath and then collapse. In the elderly, it is possible to have a 'silent' myocardial infarction with no symptoms at all.

Infarction may be diagnosed with an ECG, but not necessarily. Usually, diagnosis is retrospective, using serial ECGs and blood levels of enzymes or proteins released from the cardiac muscle when damaged. Most useful is the titre of the cardiac proteins Troponin T and I. They are specific to cardiac muscle and are released within 4 to 6 hours of muscle death; they can remain elevated for up to two weeks. The complications of MI vary, from immediate death because of acute heart failure, if a large part of the muscle infarcts, to none, if the infarct is small.

Arrhythmias can occur as a complication of MI, the commonest being ventricular fibrillation and ventricular tachycardia. These can be reversed with a direct current electric shock given with an automatic external defibrillator (AED). Pulseless electrical activity- PEA, (where the ECG shows a tracing but there is no contraction), or asystole (where there is no tracing at all), cannot be reversed with a shock.

Ventricular fibrillation (VF) is rapid, irregular and uncoordinated electrical activity in the ventricles, probably because of re-entry circuits within localised areas of the myocardium. The ECG shows a coarse irregular waveform without discernible P, QRS or T waves. Effective contraction and cardiac output cease, leading to loss of consciousness. It is often precipitated by ectopic beats or a burst of ventricular tachycardia, particularly when they are complications of acute MI. If it occurs within 48 hours of acute MI, the prognosis is better than if it occurs later when more muscle damage has occurred. Ventricular fibrillation is the commonest cause of sudden death in the community.

The success rate for resuscitation of patients who 'arrest' is low. Fewer than a quarter of those who suffer a cardiac arrest in hospital survive to go home. The most likely to survive are those where the arrest is monitored and witnessed (as they would be in a coronary care unit), where the arrest is caused by myocardial ischemia with an irritable myocardium, and where the patient is defibrillated immediately. In patients whose arrest

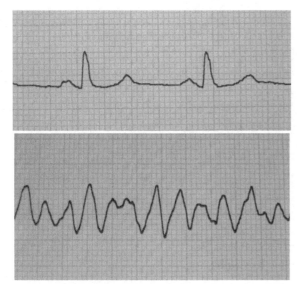

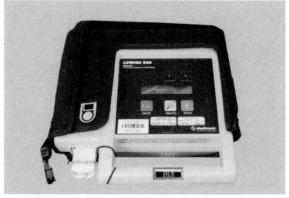

Automatic External Defibrillator (AED). This analyses the heart rhythm and advises you with audible instructions if the rhythm is 'shockable'.

Ventricular fibrillation (VF) on an ECG is obvious when compared to normal sinus rhythm at the top. This patient was being monitored on the coronary care unit when she went into VF after a myocardial infarction. Resuscitation was successful.

occurs outside the coronary care unit in unmonitored areas, it usually follows a slow progressive deterioration in their physiological well-being with hypoxaemia and hypotension. This leads to asystole or a pulseless heart, in which case the prognosis is poor. Attempts have been made to avoid this by carrying out 'Early Warning Scores' in which a patient is awarded a score on a scale depending on observation of respiratory rate, heart rate, blood pressure and level of consciousness. If a patient reaches a certain risk level, then their nurse will call the critical care outreach team or medical emergency team, depending upon the local arrangements.

Resuscitation is divided into basic and advanced life support. Basic life support can be performed by a lay person who has been trained but who has no equipment other than perhaps a pocket airway to inflate the lungs from their own mouth. Advanced life support requires equipment and specialised skills. In the hospital, there should be no such distinction; basic life support given by the first person to witness the collapse should continue seamlessly to defibrillation, if appropriate, and advanced management by the medical emergency team. After starting CPR, you would normally expect the emergency team to arrive within a few minutes. However, modern automatic defibrillators will automatically analyse the electrical

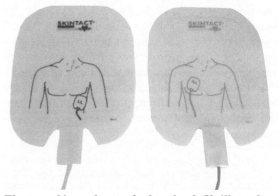

The two skin pads attached to the defibrillator have clear diagrams as to where they should be placed.

activity of the heart and decide if there is a 'shockable' rhythm.

When a patient collapses after an MI, their survival depends upon successful defibrillation with an AED. The sooner this is used, the better their chance; each minute's delay reduces their chance by 10%. If they have just collapsed, then they will have enough oxygen on board for a few minutes. You should still start with chest compression as this makes ventricular fibrillation coarser and increases the chance of a successful defibrillation.

You will find there are many resuscitation trolleys containing all the equipment throughout the hospital. This will be checked regularly, and the defibrillator tested every morning. You should make sure you are familiar with the equipment.

The chances of you having to carry out CPR are low. This makes it important that you practise on a

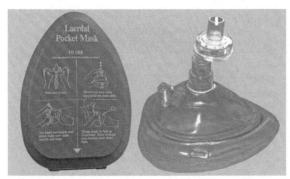

A pocket mask used for basic life support. The mask fits tightly around the mouth and nose to facilitate lung inflation without mouth contact. There is a filter on the end and a port to connect oxygen should it be available. There is guidance printed on the case.

manikin at least once every six months and know the procedure by heart so that if needed, you will be able to carry it out. Attend the resuscitation training sessions and get a certificate to prove that you have done it. CPR always gets tested in postgraduate dental examinations. This is a gift to the candidates as they all always do well, although a significant proportion do the chest compression too fast because they have not practised on a manikin recently.

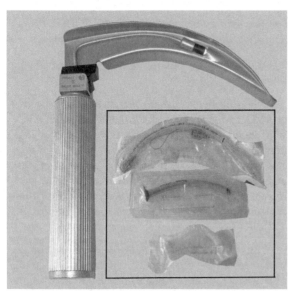

Airway management equipment is included on the resuscitation trolley. This includes the laryngoscope, endotracheal, nasopharyngeal and oral airways. You should only use the oral airway, leaving the use of the others to those trained in intubation.

The process gives a structured approach to assessment. It starts with the easiest to recognise, and most dangerous, problems which are easier to deal with and progresses to the more difficult.

A - Airway

Upper airway obstruction. If they can answer a verbal question then they are not obstructed. Caused by secretions or vomit or swelling. Tongue may be fallen back if patient not fully conscious. Stridor (wheezing on breathing out) is a sign. Lift the chin, tilt head, suction. May need anaesthetist if upper airway is obstructed.

B - Breathing

Respiratory rate is most important. Look for chest expansion, depth of breath & use of accessory muscle of respiration. Listen for wheeze from end of bed, then with stethoscope. What is their colour: are they pale or blue? Feel if the chest is expanding equally. Give them a short spell of 15L/ min. of O_2. Their saturation on pulse oximeter must be 90% at the very least.

C - Circulation

Look for pallor, anaemia or signs of blood loss. Check capillary refill time (normally < 2 secs). Feel central (carotid) pulse; if absent systolic probably <70. Feel peripheral limb temperature and peripheral pulse; if no radial pulse systolic <90. Check pulse rate & rhythm. (BP may be normal in severe hypovolaemia shock.) What is the O2 saturation & urine output? Both may be low in hypovolaemia or cardiogenic shock. If not obvious sign of heart failure assume hypovolaemia and give 200 mls fluid then reassess.

D - Disability (Neurological)

Are they conscious, alert and orientated and conversing or confused? State can be described according to the A V P U system. A – alert, V – responds to voice, P – responds to pain, U – unresponsive. Can use Glasgow Coma Scale to describe patient's condition . Measure blood glucose and nurse in supine position if unconscious.

E - Exposure (for full examination)

Expose the patient to carry out a full physical examination in more detail.

Resuscitation procedure

The aim should be to start CPR immediately, and, if appropriate, defibrillate within three minutes at the most.

The following process is based on the Resuscitation Council's recommendations for in-hospital resuscitation and makes the following assumptions: the collapse has occurred during minor oral surgery and thus includes clearing the mouth of debris or obstruction; there are other health care professionals present who can participate in the process; there is certain equipment available which would not be available in a non-hospital setting such as ECG, pulse oximetry and blood pressure monitoring; there is a medical emergency or resuscitation team available to respond to a '2222' call; there are health care professionals present with the appropriate equipment and expertise to gain intra-venous access.

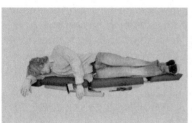

1. When you find a patient collapsed or witness a patient lose consciousness you should shout for help and check that there is nothing that will compromise your own personal safety.

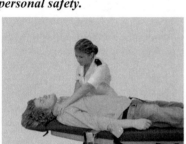

2. You should shake the patient vigorously by the shoulders and shout, asking if they are OK, to see if there is any responsiveness. If patient is responsive, see box below:

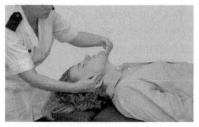

3. If no response turn patient on his back, open his airway by tilting his head back and lifting his chin forward.

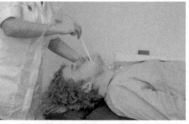

4. Check there is no obstruction in his mouth to compromise the airway; suck out if there is any debris.

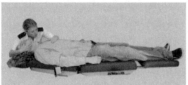

5. Listen for breathing and simultaneously look and feel for air and chest movement for 10 seconds (no longer). It is more reliable to check for respiration than attempting to feel for a pulse. If patient is responsive check carotid pulse and see box below:

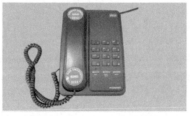

6. If there is no breathing obvious by 10 seconds ask your helper to call 'cardiac arrest' to the Medical Emergency Team by calling 2222. If you are still alone do it yourself.

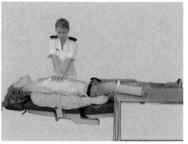

7. Start CPR by compressing the chest in the middle of the lower half of the sternum for 4 - 5 cms (about ⅓ its depth) 100 times per

---

If the patients is responsive at stage 2 or 5 above:

If it is a simple vaso-vagal syncope showing the signs described in the previous chapter and the patient recovers quickly, tip patient back, give oxygen and carry on.

Otherwise access the patient with ABCDE approach. Call medical emergency team as appropriate. Give patient oxygen through mask and monitor with a pulse oximeter, attach ECG leads attach monitor and blood pressure cuffs and take readings. Gain venous access.

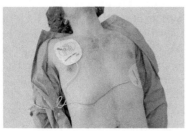

8. Put on the Automatic External Defibrillator (AED) pads in the positions shown on the pads. Do this without interrupting chest compression.

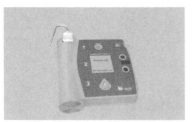

9. Plug the lead into the AED, press the on switch and follow the verbal instructions.

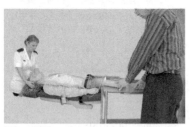

The AED, when ready, will instruct you to 'stand well clear of the patient' while it analyses the cardiac rhythm; it will tell you to shock the patient if it does not detect sinus rhythm and after further analysis of the electrical activity will tell you to start CPR again if appropriate. You should aim to defibrillate within 60 to 120 seconds; every minute's delay reduces the chance of a successful outcome by about 10%.

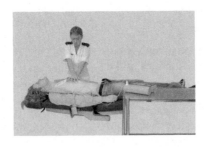

10. If the patient does not respond, and the AED tells you to, restart CPR with chest compression.

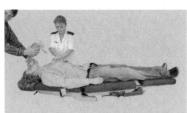

11. Now introduce ventilation using the face mask with a reservoir bag. You can place an oral airway to prevent tongue obstruction. The lungs should be ventilated with the bag over the airway for 1 second with enough volume to expand the chest as seen in normal breathing. Oxygen should be attached to the bag as soon as possible. Chest compression and ventilation should proceed at the ratio of 30:2. Chest compression is the more important.

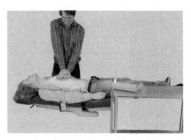

12. Change the person doing chest compression every 2 minutes to prevent fatigue. The AED will analyse the rhythm periodically and tell you to shock the patient if necessary. If you have sufficient helpers someone can place an IV line before the Medical Emergency Team arrive.

Resuscitation in examinations

For examinations you should memorise the resuscitation council's recommendations for dental practice.

This assumes no IV access skills and no expertise in feeling a carotid pulse and no 'on-site' emergency team. It relies on you calling 999 for back up.

You should practice on a manikin, in particular the rate of cardiac compression which candidates often get too fast.

You should practice lung inflation with mouth inflation and a pocket mask which is easier to get an oral air seal with than a bag and mask.

In the exam you will have to operate alone which means you will need to simulate calling for help (including dialing 999) and fetching equipment yourself before starting chest compression.

The principle is that unless you can defibrillate the patient with the automatic external defibrillator the patient will die.

18. <u>Ordering and Interpretation of Blood Tests</u>

<u>*Blood tests used in Oral & Maxillofacial Surgery*</u>

Commonly

Full blood count

• As a baseline measurement of haemoglobin in major cases where significant blood loss is expected.

• Where a patient has bled more than anticipated to check platelets.

• Occasionally if a patient has been anaemic in the past and is due for surgery under anaesthetic.

• Occasionally for a patient with stomatitis (see B12 etc. below).

INR

• Before surgery in a patient taking warfarin but check their anticoagulant card before testing.

Coagulation screen

• Where there has been inappropriate bleeding.

Urea/Electrolytes

• Diabetics and patients on diuretics before surgery under anaesthetic.

• Rarely in patients with renal disease who are due for surgery.

Glucose

• Diabetics due for surgery under anaesthetic.

• Patients who present with severe infections or unexplained candidiasis**.**

<u>*Blood tests used in Oral & Maxillofacial Surgery*</u>

Sometimes

B12, folate ferritin

• Patients with stomatitis; however, rarely abnormal and of dubious significance.

LFTs

• Patients who present with mouth cancer to check for compromised function which might be caused by metastatic disease or alcohol.

• To check for serum protein levels which might be decreased if nutrition has been compromised by difficulty with eating or high alcohol consumption.

• Patients who present with inappropriate bleeding whose liver dependent clotting factors may be reduced by alcohol or other liver disease.

<u>Occasionally</u>

Anti-nuclear antibodies and Rheumatoid factor

• If Sjögren's syndrome is suspected.

<u>Rarely</u>

E.S.R & C-reactive protein

• To monitor treatment response in severe sepsis.

C4

• As a screening test for hereditary angio-oedema.

Bone and parathyroid hormone

• Where a central giant cell granuloma is found in the jaw to exclude hyper-parathyroidism.

Ordering of tests

We will discuss the blood tests we commonly use, the basis for them, and how they may help us.

In most hospitals, requests must be made on-line; in this case, the patient will be given a printed request for the phlebotomist with a bar code or QR code for exact identification. Outpatients and inpatients whose blood tests can be anticipated may be bled by a phlebotomist, but you may have to do it yourself for urgent unplanned ward admissions if there is no clinical support worker available to do it. Where written request forms are used, they must be completed legibly and local policies conformed to regarding labelling forms and blood bottles.

Interpretation

The results will need to be interpreted intelligently and matched to the clinical problem being considered. It should be compared to the reference range which does not necessarily equate with 'normal' in every case. The individual result may be affected by the patient's age, sex, ethnicity, medication, alcohol taken or the time of day; they may also be affected by pregnancy. The reference range which relates to the range of results for a normal population; this will therefore depend upon the population being compared. 2.5% of the normal population is removed from the top and bottom ends of the reference range so that a result just outside the range does not necessarily mean the patient is abnormal. 5% of the normal population will have a result outside the reference range or 1:20. Thus, the result must be carefully considered with the patient's clinical condition and the results of other investigations.

All results should be followed up; it is unacceptable to request any investigation without looking at the results. For routine investigations, the results should be available on the hospital computer system on the same day; others may take longer. Sometimes this will be followed by a printed report which should be signed to show it has been looked at and filed in the patient's notes, but usually there will be just an electronic report on the clinical records system which is available for printing if desired. Where a result is outside the reference range, a haematologist or biochemist may look at it and make suggestions for further action or investigation.

You should only order tests which are essential for the patient's management. Not only will this avoid incurring the expense of unnecessary tests, but it will avoid the problem of trying to interpret the results that are outside the reference range, 5% of which may not represent an abnormality.

All investigations, including blood tests, should be subjected to the "so what" test before they are ordered. This means that you should be clear that the result will have some impact on the management of the patient before you tick the box on the request form or computer screen. You should be clear of the significance of a positive or negative result. Too many investigations are ordered by junior doctors without sufficient justification.

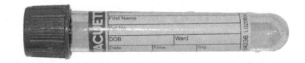

Blood for a full blood count is collected in a lavender topped colour coded bottle. It contains ethylene diamine tetra acetic acid (EDTA) which stops the sample from clotting by removing calcium ions from the plasma.

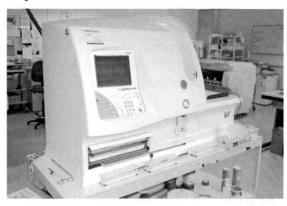

In the laboratory the full blood count is determined by one of these machines. The sample is shaken to ensure even distribution of cells and bottles are loaded in. It can process 120 samples per hour.

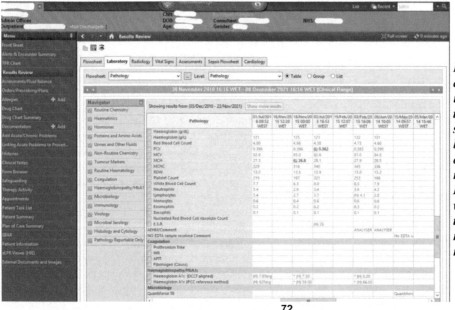

Blood test results on computer screen. You usually order tests from the clinical records system on a computer but you may have to order on a paper request form.
In the following pages we have shown some test results on paper reports, these show the reference ranges.

Haematology tests

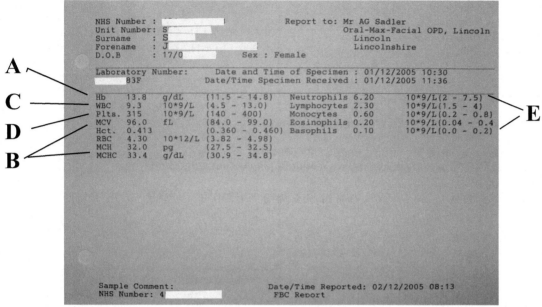

A —
C —
D —
B —

```
NHS Number  :                        Report to: Mr AG Sadler
Unit Number: S                                  Oral-Max-Facial OPD, Lincoln
Surname     : S                                 Lincoln
Forename    : J                                 Lincolnshire
D.O.B       : 17/0              Sex : Female

Laboratory Number:      Date and Time of Specimen : 01/12/2005 10:30
          83F             Date/Time Specimen Received : 01/12/2005 11:36

Hb     13.8   g/dL      (11.5 - 14.8)   Neutrophils 6.20   10*9/L(2 - 7.5)
WBC    9.3    10*9/L    (4.5 - 13.0)    Lymphocytes 2.30   10*9/L(1.5 - 4)
Plts.  315    10*9/L    (140 - 400)     Monocytes   0.60   10*9/L(0.2 - 0.8)
MCV    96.0   fL        (84.0 - 99.0)   Eosinophils 0.20   10*9/L(0.04 - 0.4)
Hct.   0.413           (0.360 - 0.460)  Basophils   0.10   10*9/L(0.0 - 0.2)
RBC    4.30   10*12/L   (3.82 - 4.98)
MCH    32.0   pg        (27.5 - 32.5)
MCHC   33.4   g/dL      (30.9 - 34.8)




Sample Comment:                  Date/Time Reported: 02/12/2005 08:13
NHS Number: 4                    FBC Report
```

E —

Full Blood Count

The most frequently used Haematology test in OMFS is the full blood count. This tells us the haemoglobin level and the quantity and proportions of the cellular component of the blood.

A. The most usual need for a full blood count (FBC) is to estimate haemoglobin, most usually as part of pre-operative assessment for anaemia or for a baseline assessment to compare with intra-operative measurements in a patient who we expect to lose a significant amount of blood. A low haemoglobin will compromise the oxygen carrying capacity of the blood, which may be important in anaesthesia and surgery for older patients. Any patient with pre-existing cardiac or respiratory disease will be more sensitive to low oxygen availability. An individual can adapt to a low haemoglobin which has been present for some time, for example, if they have 'anaemia of chronic disease', especially so if they are fairly inactive. There is therefore no absolute lower haemoglobin level at which a patient can have an anaesthetic. However, a patient who has a low haemoglobin level consequent upon recent blood loss will be much more sensitive and may have a low tolerance to exertion or even be breathless at rest. Therefore, patients who have suffered recent trauma and lost blood are more likely to benefit from having a full blood count. In practice, we request it pre-operatively for only a few of our patients but we always would for those undergoing major surgery where a significant amount of blood may be lost, such as resection of oral cancer, orthognathic surgery or a major facial injury. The National Institute of Heath & Care (NICE) has published guidelines as to which patients we should request pre-operative investigations for; this guidance looks as if it has been written by a committee and is over complicated but it is potentially useful in preventing a lot of unnecessary tests.

Occasionally we may request an FBC (together with haematinics) if we see a patient with atrophic glossitis, which may be a symptom of chronic iron deficiency anaemia and there is thought to be an association with angular cheilitis. Our experience is that requesting an FBC for patients with sore tongues or angular cheilitis produces an enormous number of normal results from the laboratory.

B. The red cell indices Mean Cell Volume (MCV), Haematocrit (Ht), Red Blood Cell Concentration (RBCC), Mean Cell Haemoglobin Concentration (MCHC) should be interpreted together. Some are not measured but are mathematically derived from the others. They can, when considered with the clinical picture, give an indication of the cause of anaemia. Anaemia with reduced MCV, MCH and MCHC is called hypochromic-microcytic. Iron deficiency anaemia and thalassaemia produce this blood picture as sometimes can 'anaemia of chronic disease'. A normal MCV and MCHC is called normocytic and normochromic anaemia. This will include most anaemias of chronic disease as well as anaemia resulting from blood loss, haemolysis and decreased RBC formation because of renal failure, aplastic and malignant disease of the marrow. A raised MCV is called macrocytic and mostly results from vitamin B12 and folate deficiency.

If the indices are abnormal, the haematologist will examine cells under a microscope as their shape and staining characteristics may help in diagnosis; this will be in the report. Anisocytosis means the red cells vary in size, Poikilocytosis, in shape. The other terms used, macro, micro and normo, you are familiar with.

An increase in the concentration of red cells may be caused by the rare condition of polycythaemia rubra vera where there is overactivity of the marrow, but it is more commonly caused as an adaption to chronic hypoxia related to lung disease and chronic smoking. A macrocytosis is often caused by excessive alcohol intake.

If haemoglobin and red cells are present in their normal absolute quantities, they may still be in reduced concentration if there is an increase in the volume of blood plasma; this may occur if a patient has been over-hydrated by intravenous fluids. Similarly, pregnancy increases plasma volume and therefore lower estimations for Hb. and RBC. If a patient is dehydrated, then a corresponding increase in concentrations may be recorded.

C. The total white cell count is commonly increased in infection, inflammation, or tissue damage. You can expect it to be increased if a patient has a large abscess, particularly if they are systemically unwell with pyrexia, after facial trauma or after major surgery. The count will return to normal as the patient recovers; occasionally serial white counts may be used to monitor recovery, but this is unusual in our clinical practice as we can observe recovery directly. The white count may also increase in any malignant disease, particularly of the bone marrow (leukaemia).

A decrease in white cells is uncommon but can occur in viral infections and when a patient is overwhelmed by acute sepsis or cancer. It can also occur because of chemotherapy. Very low levels will lead to infection from otherwise harmless bacteria and mucosal ulceration may occur. Candidiasis of the mouth is particularly associated with a low WBC.

D. Platelets, which are an essential part of haemostasis, may be decreased in numbers in aplastic anaemia, leukaemia and because of chemotherapy or radiotherapy. However, the most common cause of low platelets is autoimmune increased breakdown seen in idiopathic thrombocytopenia purpura (ITP). This may occur as a primary disease, mostly in women, or secondary to other disease processed or caused by some

---

Causes of Anaemia

1. Iron deficiency

2. Chronic inflammation or infection (anaemia of chronic disease)

3. Blood loss

4. Deficiency of B_{12} or folate

5. Deficiency of erythropoietin (most chronic renal failure)

6. Increased RBC destruction (haemolytic anaemias)

7. Marrow failure (aplastic, usually toxic drugs or radio therapy)

8. Malignant disease in marrow (leukaemia, myeloma)

---

drugs. Most usually, we will see patients with low platelets when they need dental extractions, usually because they have ITP or have recently had chemotherapy. However, platelet levels quickly recover after chemotherapy and fluctuate with ITP so the levels should be checked just beforehand. The level needs to be very low before there is a bleeding problem, usually below about $60 \times 10^9/L$.

E. The differential white cell count shows the number of the individual types of white cells in the blood. This is of infrequent use to us in OMFS. However we will briefly explain their significance. Neutrophils are the most numerous. They offer protection against bacteria and engage in phagocytosis. They are increased in acute infections, inflammation, tissue damage, where there are solid tumours and chronic myeloid leukaemia. The lymphocytes comprise 70% T – lymphocytes, which destroy infected cells, and 30% B – lymphocytes, which produce antibodies. There are also a few 'Natural Killer' cells. Lymphocytes increase in infectious mononucleosis, several other viral infections, chronic bacterial infections and several rarer diseases, which include toxoplasmosis which can present with enlarged lymph nodes in the neck. They are increased in chronic lymphatic leukaemia and non-Hodgkin's lymphoma. Monocytes phagocytose foreign material and have a role in presenting antigens to T lymphocytes; they are rarely increased in number. Eosinophils phagocytose larger foreign material and have a role in killing organisms larger than bacteria. They are present at the site of inflammation caused by allergic reactions such as allergic asthma and hay fever. They are increased in parasitic worm infections and allergic diseases, as well as occasionally in Hodgkin's lymphoma. Basophils are rarely seen in the peripheral blood. They become Mast cells in the tissues, which release mediators of acute inflammation; they are raised in chronic myeloid leukaemia, but rarely otherwise.

Coagulation Studies

Intermittently patients with a history of prolonged or excessive bleeding present needing surgery or dental extraction. The most important part of the investigation is the clinical history, but you will need to arrange a full blood count to check their platelet count and a coagulation screen.

The coagulation screen comprises three tests. Prothrombin time (PT) tests the extrinsic coagulation pathway clotting factors and the final common pathway as it forms fibrin. The activated partial thromboplastin time (APTT) assesses the intrinsic and final common pathways and the thrombin time (TT) the final pathway only. If all of these are normal, then the coagulation cascade should be normal and produce normal fibrin for haemostasis. If any are abnormal, the report will advise what to do next; to retest, do additional investigations or to refer the patient to a haematologist. If the patient is still bleeding, a haematologist's help will be needed immediately.

The most common inherited clotting defects are Haemophilia A, followed by Haemophilia B or Christmas Disease. These are caused by a deficiency of factors 8 and 9, respectively. They are part of the intrinsic pathway, so that the APTT will be prolonged, whereas PT and TT will be normal. More commonly, clotting factors are deficient due to liver disease, which is acquired. PT will be most sensitive to this, but in severe liver disease PT and APTT will both be prolonged; it is unusual for the TT to be affected.

You will come across a lot of patients taking anti-coagulants, most frequently warfarin, which has a long half-life and is taken orally. This is used to prevent clots in patients who have had a deep vein thrombosis and pulmonary embolus and as primary prevention for patients at risk for several reasons, most commonly atrial fibrillation. Heparin is used in hospital for rapid anticoagulation of patients who have thrombosis. It has to be given subcutaneously or intravenously; it has a very short half-life and is therefore easily controlled. Warfarin therapy is monitored using the PT, Heparin, with the APTT. The PT is expressed as the international normalised ratio (INR) which is the ratio of the patient's PT over the mean of the PT reference range using an international sensitivity index. This makes the result more standardised for comparison purposes.

Warfarin is the most commonly used anti-coagulant. An INR result of 2 means that the patient's blood will take twice as long to clot than the control. Patients who need anticoagulation have differing target values depending on their condition. Those who are taking it because they have atrial fibrillation or have had a recent deep vein thrombosis will have a target value of between 2 and 3 whereas those who have a mechanical heart valve replacement are at higher risk and will have a higher therapeutic range of between 3 and 4. We receive many referrals for dental extractions for patients on warfarin but it has been shown repeatedly that if the INR is below 4, then if they are managed correctly with the sockets sutured and packed with oxidised cellulose gauze, then post extraction bleeding is no more of a problem than patients not on warfarin. If the INR is above 4, then this is outside the therapeutic range and the patients should see their GP to have their dose adjusted before the extractions.

Erythrocyte Sedimentation Rate and C Reactive Protein

Erythrocyte sedimentation rate (ESR) is a simple test in which anti-coagulated blood is left for the red cells to sediment to the bottom of a tube. The result is expressed in the number of millimetres the red cells fall in an hour. The ESR will be increased in disease processes that increase certain plasma proteins, which cause aggregation of the red cells and in certain anaemias where the number of red cells is decreased. ESR is normally 1 – 10 mm/hour in males and 5-10 mm/hour in females. This increases with age by about 0.8 mms per 5 years. ESR is a very unspecific test; it is raised in pregnancy, where there is significant tissue damage, infection, malignancy and in certain individuals with no disease. A decrease in ESR is uncommon and usually of little clinical significance; it occurs in polycythaemia.

C reactive protein (CRP) is present normally in low concentration in the plasma and is a more modern non-specific test as an alternative to ESR. It is increased in inflammation, infection and malignancy, but is not affected by red cell numbers.

ESR and CRP are used to monitor treatment responses to patients with complicated and extensive disease processes, e.g. inflammatory or infective.

Biochemistry tests

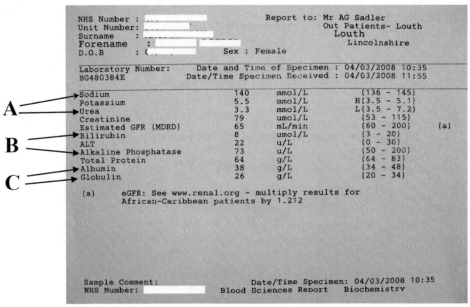

```
NHS Number :                        Report to: Mr AG Sadler
Unit Number:                                   Out Patients- Louth
Surname    :                                   Louth
Forename   :                                   Lincolnshire
D.O.B      :                Sex : Female

Laboratory Number:      Date and Time of Specimen : 04/03/2008 10:35
BG480384E               Date/Time Specimen Received : 04/03/2008 11:55

Sodium                  140     mmol/L      (136 - 145)
Potassium               5.5     mmol/L      H(3.5 - 5.1)
Urea                    3.3     mmol/L      L(3.5 - 7.2)
Creatinine              79      umol/L      (53 - 115)
Estimated GFR (MDRD)    65      mL/min      (60 - 200)      (a)
Bilirubin               8       umol/L      (3 - 20)
ALT                     22      u/L         (0 - 30)
Alkaline Phosphatase    73      u/L         (50 - 200)
Total Protein           64      g/L         (64 - 83)
Albumin                 38      g/L         (34 - 48)
Globulin                26      g/L         (20 - 34)

(a)     eGFR: See www.renal.org - multiply results for
        African-Caribbean patients by 1.212


Sample Comment:             Date/Time Specimen: 04/03/2008 10:35
NHS Number:                 Blood Sciences Report    Biochemistry
```

Labels on left: A (pointing to Urea), B (pointing to Bilirubin), C (pointing to Globulin)

Urea and Electrolytes

A. Urea and electrolytes (Us & Es) Sodium (Na^+), and Potassium (K^+) have been traditionally requested and analysed together. Nowadays, however, the analysing equipment will process multiple biochemical and immunological assays simultaneously on one sample.

Na^+ is the primary electrolyte in the blood; hypernatraemia may be due to a very high salt intake or dehydration from inadequate fluid intake or excessive fluid loss from sweating or diarrhoea. Na^+ concentration may be low in excessive fluid retention. Neither of these situations are of much relevance to us in every day OMFS where, should we encounter patients with severe electrolyte or fluid balance abnormality, we would request the assistance of a physician.

Hyperkalaemia may be due to renal disease or diabetes. Hypokalaemia may be due to excessive K^+ loss in diarrhoea or from excessive loss due to diuretic medication. As surgeons our main concern with abnormal K^+ concentration will be the potential effect on cardiac muscle. Severe hyperkalaemia can result in instability of the cardiac muscle, leading to cardiac arrest, and in hypokalaemia cardiac arrhythmias may occur. We would therefore wish to test for K^+ concentration for any patient receiving a general anaesthetic if they have renal disease, poorly controlled diabetes or are taking diuretics. In general, a narrow reference range for a blood test indicates potentially serious consequences when it is either too high or low and this is the case with potassium.

Urea is a waste product of normal metabolism. There is a gradual increase in the blood concentration with age due to a gradual decline of renal function. Urea may be increased in more advanced renal disease but not early on. It may also be increased in starvation and dehydration.

Creatinine is a waste product, more specifically of muscle metabolism. Raised creatinine will be a more sensitive marker for early renal disease.

Estimated Glomerular Filtration Rate (eGFR) is calculated from the MDRD (Modification of Diet in Renal Disease study) formula; this includes creatinine level, age, sex and ethnicity. If the estimated glomerular filtration rate (eGFR) is decreased, further investigation may be needed for chronic kidney disease. If a low eGFR is found on routine testing, we should alert the patient's GP to deal with this later.

B. Bilirubin, alanine transferase (ALT) and alkaline phosphatase are together known as the liver function tests (LFTs). Bilirubin is derived from haemoglobin breakdown and is increased in liver disease, where there is obstruction to bile flow and in haemolytic anaemias where there is increased breakdown of red cells. If it is very high, the patient may be clinically jaundiced. Alanine transferase and alkaline phosphatase are metabolic catalysts in liver cells. They are released into the bloodstream, where they have no function, when liver cells are damaged and hence their presence usually indicates liver disease. However, they are present in other tissues, notably the pancreas, kidney, heart and muscle. Alkaline phosphatase is present in osteoclasts and will be released into the plasma in any condition where there is high osteoclastic activity. This will include childhood growth spurts, Paget's disease of bone, healing fractures and bone cancer, including metastatic disease. We may therefore wish to order these tests when a patient has a history of liver disease and is to receive an anaesthetic or if they have cancer and we want to know if metastatic disease has affected liver function or we wish to know if there might be bone involvement.

C. Albumin and globulin together make up the plasma proteins. Albumin is the more abundant, being about 60%; it is synthesised in the liver from amino acids. It acts as a transport medium for water insoluble substances in the blood and is important in maintaining blood plasma volume. Albumin may be low in chronic liver disease (cirrhosis) but not in acute; this will lead to increased fluid in the interstitial spaces and possibly oedema. It may be reduced in malnutrition due to inadequate amino acid intake or in severe burns. It will be raised in patients who are dehydrated. We will want to know the albumin level for new patients who present with advanced mouth cancer, as they may have a low albumin from inadequate nutrition. Globulins make up the rest of the plasma proteins; they include the gamma globulins, which are antibodies, and they act as enzymes and carriers. They may be elevated in chronic infections and renal disease and may be decreased in renal disease, which leads to protein loss, haemolytic anaemia, liver disease and hypogammaglobulinaemia.

Immunology tests

These are used infrequently in OMFS. However, we may occasionally test for antinuclear antibodies (ANA) in a patient with a dry mouth who we suspect may have Sjögren's syndrome (SS). ANA are raised in a variety of conditions, such as systemic lupus, rheumatoid arthritis and chronic active hepatitis. About 70% of patients with SS will have raised titres of ANA. These are expressed as the dilution at which they may be detected; normal is 1:40. In addition, 70% of SS patients will have a raised titre of the ANA sub types anti-SS-A (also known as anti-Ro) and 40% will have a raised titre of anti-SS-B (known as anti-La). Rheumatoid factor is also likely to be raised in 60% of these patients. The significance of SS (apart from the dry mouth) is that there is an increased incidence of low grade lymphoma and this may be associated with a low level of complement C4.

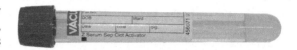

Combined clinical chemistry and immunology is tested on serum. Blood is taken into a tube which contains a gel, with silica in it; this activates coagulation. The tube is centrifuged to separate the serum; the gel moves up forming a barrier between serum and fibrin

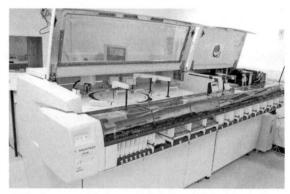

This integrated general chemistry & immunoassay analyser will process 1200 clinical chemistry and 200 immunoassays per hour. Only one serum specimen is needed for both.

Immunoglobulins may be tested in patients who have repeated infections. IgM will be raised in patients who have significant acute inflammation. IgE may be of help in supporting a diagnosis of an allergy. However, the normal range is very wide, and it is possible to have a raised specific IgE against a single allergen when total IgE is normal; thus, it is of limited use. Occasionally we see a patient with recurrent oedematous swelling around the face. A rare cause of this is hereditary angio-oedema due to complement C1 inhibitor deficiency. Patients with these clinical symptoms should have their complement C4 tested as a screening test. If this is normal, then they will not have heredity angio-oedema and there is no need to test for complement C1 inhibitor levels.

19. <u>Venepuncture</u>

You may be called upon to bleed patients for haematological, biochemical or immunological testing or to place intravenous cannulae to be used to deliver parenteral fluids or medication.

Taking a Blood Sample

The need for you to bleed patients will depend upon the availability of phlebotomists. In some hospitals, they carry out this task not only for outpatients who need investigations but do a round of the wards each morning. To avail yourself of this service, you will need to make an on-line request or write a request card the night before or early in the morning before they arrive. Similarly, intravenous catheters may be placed by clinical support workers, but this may not be the case in many establishments, so if there are none, or they are not around, the task may fall on you.

Venepuncture will be a useful skill to learn if you are ever going to work when you will give intravenous sedation. Your hospital appointment will give you ample opportunity to learn and become practised.

Before you start, prepare yourself by learning what equipment you need, how to use it and how to select suitable veins. You should be organised and practise on a manikin before starting on patients. The operating theatre is an ideal place to get practice as the anaesthetist will put an IV cannula into every patient having an anaesthetic and most will be happy to teach and supervise you.

The Closed Vacuum system

There are several commercially available closed systems for taking blood. They have several advantages over using a hypodermic syringe and needle. The main one is that the blood goes straight into the collecting bottle without the need to decant it, leading to less risk of spillage and injury from the needle.

However, a hypodermic needle and syringe may still be the easiest way of bleeding a patient if they have small or otherwise difficult veins, such as might be the case if they have been damaged by a drug abuse habit.

All equipment for intravenous access is colour coded. A green needle (21 gauge) is the smallest that can be used to take blood samples. A smaller needle will cause the blood to haemolyse (damage to the cell walls leading to release of their contents into the plasma). This will give inaccurate results, particularly for haemoglobin or potassium.

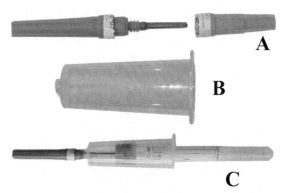

Here is a 21 gauge needle with a valve (A), a hollow plastic tube that the needle screws onto (B), and a vacuumed blood sample bottle (C). This has a rubber bung on the end which is inserted into the tube after the needle has been inserted into the vein. Blood flows into the tube, encouraged by the vacuum. The vacuum is such that flow stops when there is sufficient blood. The valve allows the bottle to be removed while the needle is still in the vein without spillage so that another tube can be attached for a different test.

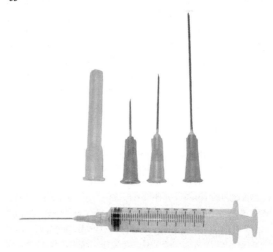

Hypodermic needles and syringe for venepuncture

When using a syringe to take blood, you should be careful to withdraw the plunger only gently and not squirt the blood out quickly through the needle, which will also cause haemolysis.

The smaller needles (blue 23 gauge and orange 25 gauge) should only be used for injecting medication; they are too small for taking blood. The larger the gauge number, the smaller is the outside diameter of the needle.

Choosing a vein

When finding a vein, the arm should be compressed by a tourniquet, a blood pressure cuff or by an assistant. The pressure applied should be between systolic and diastolic blood pressure so that arterial blood will flow into the arm, but venous flow out is occluded. The vein will be encouraged to stand out if it is warm, if the patient's hand is repeatedly made into a fist to pump the blood, and if the vein is tapped gently with your hand.

First, choose a vein that can be seen and can be felt. If there are none, your second choice is one that can be felt but not seen. A vein that can be seen but not felt should be your last choice, but it will be difficult. An elderly person may have veins that can be easily felt but are difficult to cannulate and withdraw blood from.

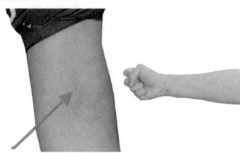 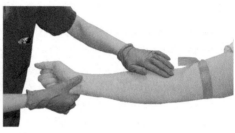

The ante-cubital fossa is the best site for taking blood from adults.

Ask the patient to repeatedly make a fist which encourages blood flow so that the vein stands out more.

Tapping the vein with your finger will also encourage it to be prominent.

Equipment needed for taking blood

Trolley
Sharps bin
A high sided tray for equipment
A paper towel or pad to absorb any spilt blood
PPE (gloves and apron) x 2

Hand sanitizer
Chlorhexidine wipes for trolley and tray
Disposable tourniquet
Chlorhexidine wipe for skin
Blood bottles and request form as appropriate
Cotton wool swab and tape to secure it to skin

Venepuncture Preparation (away from patient)

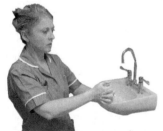

1. Decontaminate Hands

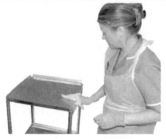

3. Clean trolley with alcohol wipe

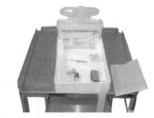

5. Equipment collected in tray on trolley ready to take to patient

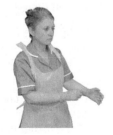

2. Put on PPE

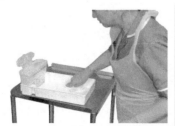

4. Clean inside of tray

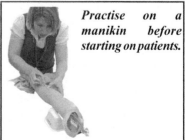

Practise on a manikin before starting on patients.

Venepuncture procedure

1. *Introduce yourself*

2. *Identify patient by name, date of birth and hospital number*

3. *On the patient, check any in-patient identity band against hospital records.*

4. *Explain what you intend to do and why.*

5. *Explain side-effects (bruising bleeding discomfort etc).*

6. *Ask about any medical history possible complications, e.g. bleeding problem, latex allergy.*

7. *Ask if they have has samples taken before. Enquire about any preferred veins for sampling.*

8. *Make patient comfortable supporting arm.*

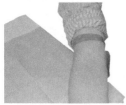

9. *Apply tourniquet and identify vein.*

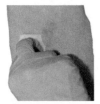

10. *Clean the skin over the vein with a disposable alcohol wipe.*

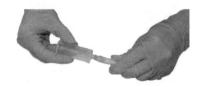

11. *Screw the needle onto the hub.*

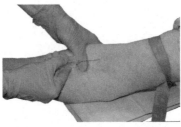

12. *Apply traction to skin below and to side of vein to immobilize the vein.*

13. *Advance needle through skin and into vein bevel up at about 30 degrees.*

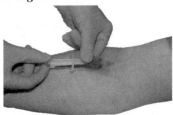

14. *Release traction when needle is in the vein, push the vacuumed specimen tube into the hub so that it engages with the needle valve; the required amount of blood will flow into the bottle.*

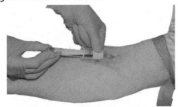

15. *If you need another sample for a different test remove the bottle and replace it with another.*

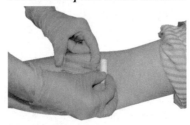

16. *Remove the last bottle, release the tourniquet then remove the needle while applying pressure with cotton wool, tape the cotton wool down.*

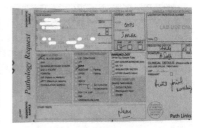

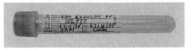

17. *Place the needle in the sharps box and clean up the equipment, remove gloves and de-contaminate hands.*

18. *Fill in request form and label the bottle or make request on-line through patient records system as appropriate for your hospital. If your hospital used electronic requests you may have to print a bar code to stick on the specimen bottle. Always print patient's full name on requests and bottles. Document in patients notes. Place specimens in transport bag to go to laboratory.*

If, after two attempts, you have failed to get blood should withdraw from the field of battle and retire to regroup. If the patient is in pain, passed out, or worse still making jokes at your expense, if he is covered with blood or there is a pile of bloodstained swabs or blood in the bed sheets then it is time to give up and ask someone else to do it.

However, if you have maintained your dignity without causing a mess, then blame the patient's awkward veins and consider your options. Tidy up, throw away the used sharps and swabs and, if you consider you have a reasonable chance of success, permit yourself one (but only one) further attempt before asking someone else to do it.

The Venflon winged intravenous cannula

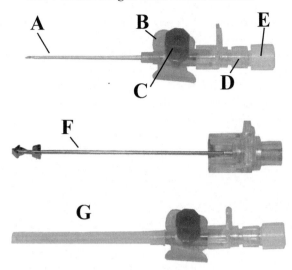

The venflon consists of a plastic cannula (A), with wings, (B), to facilitate attachment to the skin. There is a side port (C) for attachment of a syringe to administer intravenous medication. The cannula has a port at the end (D) which can be capped (E) or used to attach an intravenous giving set. The catheter is mounted on a needle (F) which protrudes from the end of the plastic cannula for venepuncture. When the needle is removed from the plastic cannula a safety device attached to the sharp end is activated. The assembled venflon (G) comes mounted within a protective plastic sheath.

Choosing a vein

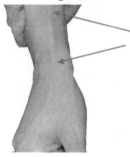 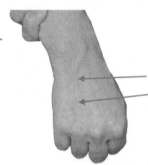

Veins on the lateral side of the wrist are very suitable for IV drips (use the non-dependent arm). It can be painful but a small bleb of local anaesthetic (without vasoconstrictor) adjacent to the vein will be helpful.

However, the back of the hand is used more often for cannulae used for medication.

Colour Coding for Cannulae

Colour	Gauge size	Used for
Blue	22G	Crystalloid
Pink	20G	Crystalloid & Colloid
Green	18G	Crystalloid, colloid & blood
Grey	16G	Crystalloid, colloid & blood
Orange	14G	Crystalloid, colloid & blood

Cannulae are coded according to gauge size. The larger the size of the catheter, the more easily fluid can pass through it. The minimum size for giving fluids would be a 22 gauge (colour coded blue) and the minimum size for giving blood products would be an 18 (colour green). A larger gauge 16 (coloured grey) is more reliable & a 14 (coloured orange) would be best. The most commonly used sizes for adults are 20 (pink) and 18 (green).

Equipment needed for cannulation

Cannula pack (see illustration) and correct size cannula
Disposable tourniquet
Sharps bin
Tray
5 to 10 mls of 0.9% saline flush
smallest cannula needed for the task (giving IV fluids or medication).

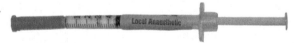

In addition you may like to use some 2% plain lignocaine (not with vasoconstrictor) drawn into a syringe with a small gauge needle. This may be placed into the skin adjacent to the vein to make the process more comfortable for the patient.

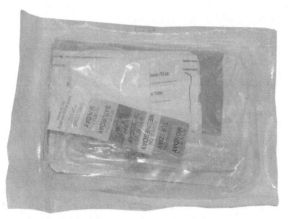

Cannulation Pack

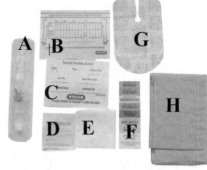

A: venflon bivalve cannula B: VIP score card (Visual Infusion Phlebitis: a score of 2 indicates the cannula should be replaced i.e. 2 of pain, swelling or erythema.) C: placement record label D: alcohol wipe E: sterile swabs F: day review labels G: dressing H: sterile drape

Cannulation procedure

1. Clean hands, put on gloves, place sterile towel beneath patient's hand to create a sterile field.

2. Introduce yourself, identify patient, explain and get verbal consent as for venepuncture

3. Position patient comfortably

4. Find suitable vein.

5. Apply tourniquet 10 cms above.

6. Palpate straight rebounding vein.

7. Release tourniquet.

8. Open cannula pack onto the tray.

9. Ensure clinical waste bin or bag is available.

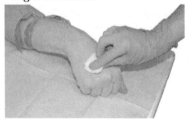

11. Clean skin with alcohol or chlorhexidine wipe for 30 seconds and allow to dry.

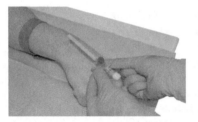

12. Straighten the cannula wings.

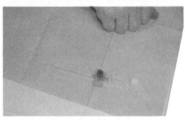

13. Remove the bung and place along with cannula on sterile towel.

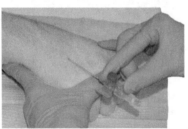

14. Remove the needle cover from the cannula, stabilize the vein by stretching the skin over the vessel with your thumb. Insert the needle through the skin and into the vein with the bevel up at an angle of 15 to 30 degrees.

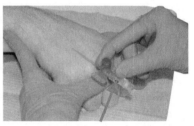

15. As soon as the first flash back is seen lower the cannula so that it is parallel to the arm. Advance further 1 to 2 mms.

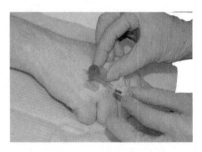

16. Withdraw the needle 2 to 3 mms and observe a second flashback long the length of the cannula. Release the tourniquet and advance the cannula fully into the vein.

17. Apply pressure to the vein above the insertion site with your forefinger.

18. Secure the cannula with your thumb and remove and dispose of the needle into the sharps bin.

19. Attach the white bung to the cannula.

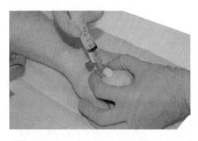

20. Flush with 5 mls saline and ask patient to report any discomfort and observe for any resistance, these would indicate that the cannula is misplaced. Dispose of the flush.

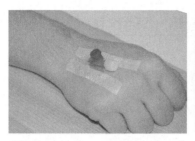

21. Secure the cannula using 2

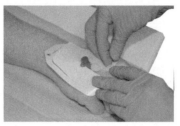

22. Apply dressing.

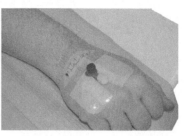

23. Apply label to dressing with initials of person siting the cannula and date and time of insertion.

24. Dispose of gloves and apron.

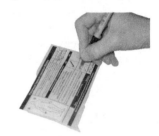

26. Fill in IV form and apply cannula produce sticker if available, record the date time site and name and status of person siting the cannula.

27. Document in patient's notes.

20. <u>Prescribing Medication in the Hospital</u>

When you work in the hospital, you will have to prescribe a few medications which will be unfamiliar to you and use the computerised clinical records system or prescription forms on paper that will be unfamiliar. However, the number of drugs that we use in OMFS is small. This is, of course, apart from drugs for inpatients that they have been taking prior to their hospital admission.

You will almost certainly find that the team you work for has a policy concerning which drugs to use. If not, there will be a normal accepted practice that you will soon get used to. You should prescribe only a few drugs you will become familiar with. Always check in the British National Formulary (BNF) when you first use a medication and subsequently, if you are uncertain about interactions with medication, the patient may already be taking.

You cannot prescribe any drug you like. There will be a hospital formulary of drugs that have been approved for use in the hospital. In most hospitals, this can be accessed, like all hospital policies and procedures, on the intranet. Every hospital trust will have a drug and therapeutics committee which manages the introduction of new drugs. Their approvals come from recommendations from consultants after consideration of evidence of efficacy from the literature, cost and availability of other medication with the same purpose. The committee will probably follow the recommendations of the National Institute for Heath & Care Excellence (NICE).

Outpatient scripts should be on a standard hospital outpatient prescription form which must be taken to the hospital pharmacy to be dispensed. You may find that you can only issue a script for the minimal medication needed before the patient can get to their GP for a repeat prescription. This is because the GPs hold the funding for outpatient medication.

In the unlikely event that you need to prescribe a controlled drug, you should specify the generic name of the drug, the dose, total quantity in words and figures. If using an addressograph label, sign it to prevent a new one being put on top of it. Add your signature and print your name.

Prescribing for inpatients should be on the standard inpatient prescription charts, which comprise a folder with four pages or on-line on the hospital intranet. There is a different page for drugs given once only, regular medication and drugs to be given only when

Outpatient prescribing will be very similar to what you are already used to. You should clearly indicate the identity of the drug using the generic name, the dose, route of administration, frequency and duration.

needed. There will be additional charts for prescribing intravenous fluids, insulin, anticoagulants, as well as charts for drugs administered by a syringe driver. Also, total parenteral nutrition which you will not be involved with.

Many patients coming into hospital will already be on some medication; this needs to be prescribed on the chart. The patient and medication will be assessed by the nurse and most will be able to take their own drugs themselves without having to have them dispensed by the nurse. This is called Self-Administered Medication.

Other medication will be dispensed by the patient's nurse at standard times and she will sign on the patient's chart to show that it has been given. Note that the times on the charts do not exactly fit into a

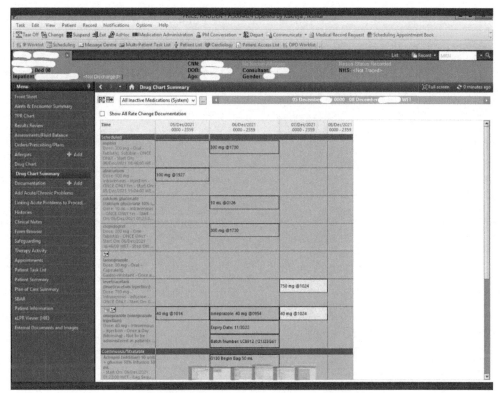

A prescription form on the clinical records system

convenient division of the day into 6 or 8 hours for drugs given x4 or x3 per day; but represents a working compromise.

Each day, a pharmacist will visit the ward and check each patient's drug chart. They will ensure that the medication is in stock in the ward drug cabinet and in sufficient quantity. They will also check the dose, frequency of administration and any interactions with other medication. This is a valuable service, as it provides a safeguard in the prevention of errors.

Antibiotic prescribing should be kept to the absolute minimum in order to reduce antimicrobial resistance, particularly MRSA and Clostridium Difficile. Every hospital will have an antibiotic policy which should be followed. For example, you may have to get the permission of a consultant microbiologist before you can prescribe a cephalosporin, if a patient is allergic to penicillin.

Antibiotics should only be prescribed for a maximum of five days, except for certain specific infections. Strictly speaking, they should be prescribed after the infecting organism has been identified by sampling and culturing and the antibiotic sensitivity defined in the laboratory. However, in practice, it may be the case that we need to prescribe before this is

known and by the time the result is expected, the need has passed and the antibiotic can be stopped. The mere presence of an infection is not necessarily an indication for antibiotics. Most oral infection, particularly of dental origin, will be adequately managed by removing the cause, draining pus and allowing the patient's immune system to deal with the rest.

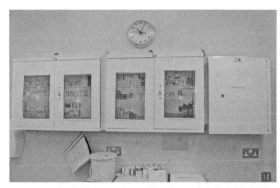

Stock drug cabinets in the treatment room on the ward. The contents are displayed by a photograph on the door. There is a separate cabinet for controlled drugs and a paper copy of the hospital formulary to refer to.

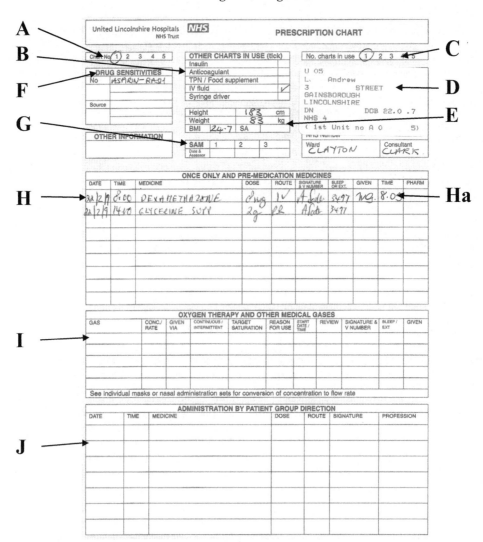

A: The number of this particular chart (Patients in hospital for a while may have accumulated several consecutive charts.) **B:** Special charts that may be in use **C:** Total number of charts in use for this patient (Usually there is only one.) **D:** Demographic details of the patient, addressograph label, ward and consultant details **E:** Height, weight, body mass index and surface area. This may have a bearing on drug dosage. **F:** Known drug allergies and sensitivities **G:** Self administered medication, number of medications the patient takes themselves and who has assessed their capability to do this and the date **H:** Prescription for drugs given once only rather than those taken on a recurring basis **Ha:** Signed and timed by nurse when drug is given **I:** Oxygen and gases. We are very unlikely to use this unless we have a patient with severe chronic obstructive pulmonary disease (COPD) or a bad post-operative chest infection. **J:** Drugs prescribed by nurses under a 'group direction' where they are permitted to prescribe certain drugs in certain circumstances according to a protocol.

Ward drug chart Page 2 & 3 of 4 (part). Regular prescriptions

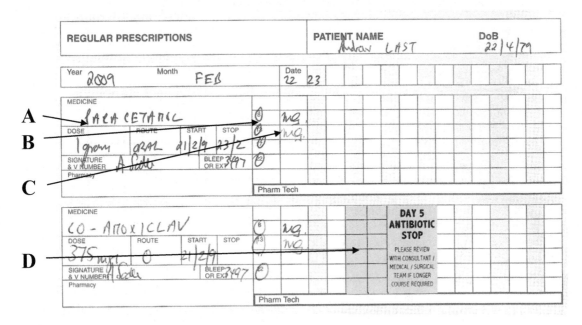

A **B** **C** **D**

REGULAR PRESCRIPTIONS					PATIENT NAME Andrew LAST		DoB 22/4/79	

Year 2009	Month FEB	Date 22	23					

A: The prescribed drug, route of administration, start & stop date, the signature of the prescriber & contact bleep or extension number for the pharmacist to contact them if there is any problem **B:** Standard times of drug rounds for the medication to be given **C:** Signature of nurse when dose given **D:** 5 day stop sticker placed by the pharmacist. This is placed automatically so that antibiotics are not continued beyond the minimum time needed.

Ward drug chart. As Required prescriptions

A **B** **C**

AS REQUIRED MEDICINES				PATIENT NAME Andrew LAST		DoB 22/4/79	

A: The prescribed drug, its reason for use, signature of the prescriber & contact bleep or extension number **B:** Dose, route, frequency it can be administered and maximum dose in 24 hours **C:** Signature of nurse when dose given, dose and time.

87

21. <u>Prescribing Fluid and Blood Replacement</u>

Humans can last only a few days without adequate water intake. The consequence of dehydration may include headache, hypotension, dizziness, fainting, delirium, loss of consciousness, and ultimately, death. Signs of dehydration will include dryness of the mouth, loss of skin elasticity, decreased or no urine output (should be 60 ml. per hour), hypotension on standing, and increased cardiac and respiratory rate.

In OMFS, we frequently need to give fluid intravenously for patients unable to take it by mouth. Usually this is because they are having surgery for which they need to be starved. Sometimes we see patients who are dehydrated; most commonly, this is because they have been drinking alcohol (which is a diuretic) and have sustained a broken jaw.

The other fluid which our patients may need replacing is blood. This may be due to heavy blood loss in trauma, but more usually is likely to be because of loss during surgery. Inadequate blood volume is called hypovolaemia, the symptoms may be nausea, thirst and dizziness. Signs may be increased pulse, decreased blood pressure and decreased peripheral perfusion, which is seen as delayed capillary refill on pressing the skin. Eventually, there may be confusion, loss of consciousness, heart failure, and death. It is unusual for OMF surgeons to administer blood

Compartment	Vol. in 70 kg. man	Na+	K+	
Intracellular	30 L	low	high	Insulin drives K into cells
Interstitial	9 L	high	low	
Intravascular	3 L	high	low	Higher protein than interstitial + blood cells

Fluid compartment properties

themselves as the acutely injured patient will already have been dealt with by the Accident and Emergency doctors, and during surgery, it will be given by the anaesthetist. However, it will do no harm to know the principles.

Types of fluid

There are basically three types of fluids which can be transfused intravenously; these are crystalloids, colloids and blood products, which are usually given as 'packed' red cells. Crystalloids are of low molecular

Crystalloids Hartman's solution and normal saline

Input	Amount (mls)	Loss	Amount (mls)
Oral fluid	1300	Urine	1500
		Stools	200
In food	900	Lungs	300
Oxidation	300	Skin	500
Total	2500	Total	2500

Daily fluid input and loss average 70kg. male

Fluid	Property	Distributes	Use
5% Glucose	Isotonic with plasma. Glucose is metabolised so is effectively just water	Distributed throughout whole body-water	Crystalloid. Provides fluid & nothing else
Hartman's solution (compound sodium lactate)	Isotonic, is water with Na^+ K^+ Ca^{++} Cl^- & Lactic acid	As above	Crystalloid. Provides fluid & electrolytes, more physiological
0.9% NaCl (normal saline)	Contains 150 mmols/L Na^+	Throughout extracellular fluid only as Na^+ is excluded from intracellular fluid	Crystalloid. Provides fluid and Na^+
Hydrolysed gelatin solutions (e.g. Gelofusine®, Haemaccel®)	High molecular weight gelatin which is metabolised & excreted over a few hours. Contains Na^+ Cl^- OH^- Anaphylaxis can occur	Initially stays in vascular compartment but is distributed into extracellular fluid as gelatin is metabolised	Colloid, expands plasma volume after blood loss
Hydroxyethyl starch (Voluven®)	High molecular weight starch, is metabolised but less quickly than gelatin. Contains Na^+ Cl^- OH^-	Stays in vascular compartment but longer than gelatin.	Colloid, expands plasma volume after blood loss. Less allergenic than gelatin
Blood	Packed cells collected from donated blood. Only fluid which carries O_2	Only in vascular compartment	Loss of blood where Hb is dropping significantly

Commonly used IV fluids (there are many others especially those used in special situations)

weight; they pass freely across cell membranes and, when given intravenously, will pass from the intravascular to interstitial fluid and then into cells. Crystalloids are cheap and without side effects; examples include dextrose solution, normal saline and Hartman's solution (which is preferred by physicians because it is more physiological). The dextrose in the solutions is of no nutritional value; it is there to make the water isotonic. Crystalloids are what we give our patients who cannot take fluid by mouth for whatever reason. It will also be the first fluid given to patients who have lost blood before colloid is given. A special note about normal (isotonic) saline: it will pass from the blood into the interstitial space but will largely be kept out of the intracellular space because Na^+ is actively pumped out in exchange for K^+.

Colloids are of high molecular weight; they do not dissolve or pass easily through cell membranes. Colloids can be used when the intravascular fluid needs replacement consequent upon blood loss. They can increase osmotic pressure and may leak across membranes causing oedema, and occasionally, they cause anaphylactic reactions. They include gelatin and starch. Gelatins are the most frequently used colloids (Haemaccel® & Gelofusine®). The colloids, because of their higher molecular weight, will stay in the intravascular compartment until the gelatin or starch is metabolised. When gelatin is metabolised, within a few hours, the fluid will then move from the intravascular compartment into the interstitial and eventually intracellular space. However, starches (Voluven®) take about 17 days to be metabolised rather than the few hours taken by gelatin, so the fluid stays in the vessels longer. Starch is therefore becoming more popular, and it is thought to provoke fewer anaphylactic reactions.

Blood

Blood (packed cells) will remain in the vessels. The reason for giving it rather than colloid is to

INTRAVENOUS FLUID CHART

United Lincolnshire Hospitals NHS
NHS Trust

Chart No.	1 2 3 4 5		No. charts in use 1 2 3 4 5				...AILS

Notes:
1. Bolus intravenous injections should be prescribed on the main drug chart.
2. If an additive is to be used are you sure that:
   it needs to be given intravenously
   it is compatible with the fluid
3. If no additive is required strike through, or write 'NIL'

DRUG SENSITIVITIES

No	✓
Source	
Height	182 cm	Weight	81 kg
BSA	m²	BMI	

Na: U ı   57
M   i
Da: 14 ı   ROAD
NEWARK
Ho: NOTTINGHAMSHIRE
NG: DOB 0ι   .87
NH: NHS 60

Ward CLAYTON   Consultant SAYLEE

			PRESCRIPTION						ADMINISTRATION					
Date	Start time	Intravenous fluid	Volume	Additive & dose	Duration infusion	Rate	Signature V Number & bleep / ext.	Date started	Time started	Started by	Checked by	Time finished	Volume given
6/9/08	22.00	5% dextrose	1 l		8 hrs		Hade.	6/9	22.05	Je	Sw	06.00	1 l
7/9/0	6.00	5% dextrose	1 l		8 hrs		Hade.	7/9	6.00	Je			
7/9/0	16.00	Normal saline	1 l		d		A Sodley						

Fluid Prescription Chart. Each bag of fluid is prescribed sequentially. The boxes on the right are for the nurse to record that it has been given. This is a suitable regime for a 24 hour period for a fit adult who is taking no fluid by mouth. Increase the amount to a litre every 6 hours if they are dehydrated (as from drinking alcohol) or pyrexial. If too much fluid is given it will be passed harmlessly as urine. Do not give fluid fast to an elderly patient or someone with heart disease as it could tip them into cardiac failure. If after two days the patient is still taking fluids IV then add 40 mols. of K^+ to each bag in the additive column.

maintain the oxygen carrying capacity of the blood. Blood transfusion has many potential complications and side effects, which include mild transfusion reactions (common), severe haemolytic reactions, sepsis, HIV or hepatitis transmission and lung injury. We therefore keep transfusion to a minimum. During surgery, depending upon the fitness of the patient, generally half of the blood volume can be lost before it is necessary to transfuse with blood.

Replacing blood loss

Blood loss is initially replaced with crystalloid (usually Hartman's solution) and then colloid; we use starch (*Voluven*®). The haemoglobin level is then monitored during surgery using a haemoglobin analyser (*HemoCue*®) and transfusion started when the level drops significantly. The haemoglobin level at which transfusion is started will depend upon several factors, which include the patient's pre-operative level, their age and cardiovascular fitness. For a fit person with a normal pre-operative level, it can drop to 8 or even lower, but in an elderly person with ischaemic heart disease, a safer level will be about 10.

So, having discussed the theory, what of prescribing fluids for patients on the ward? If you read a textbook of medicine or surgery, you will find that it can be very complicated. Fluid replacement will depend upon what fluid may have been lost and how. It may be lost as a result of vomiting, diarrhoea, blood loss, renal disease, exudates from burns, etc. It will also depend upon the amount lost, as recorded on a fluid balance chart, and the patient's renal function. However, in OMFS, we are usually dealing with patients who are generally fit and have normal kidneys; this makes it very simple.

IV fluid use in OMFS

The most likely, if not the only, circumstance in which you will be asked to prescribe fluid will be for a patient who cannot take fluid by mouth. They will

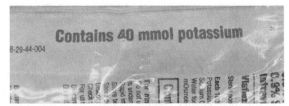

Fluid bags are available with potassium added

need only water, so you will need to write up only a crystalloid. Thus, you can prescribe a dextrose solution and add some saline for their daily Na$^+$ needs (approx. 120 to 140 mmols. per day). In the unlikely event that the patient needs fluids for more than two days, you should add some K$^+$ (approx. 60 mmols. per day). Prescribe as on the fluid chart illustrated. If the patient is dehydrated from drinking alcohol or is pyrexial (which leads to a greater insensible fluid loss), increase the amount; they will come to no harm if you give a little too much as they will pass it off as urine. However, if you have an elderly patient with a compromised heart, you could put them into heart failure if too much fluid is given too rapidly. If prescribing fluid in the emergency situation you should start with Hartman's solution or saline, as rehydrating a patient with dextrose or dextrose saline carries a risk of producing hyponatraemia, which can be dangerous. The electrolytes should normally be checked daily for a patient on IV fluids.

Use of blood for OMFS

The most commonly used blood products are packed red cells, platelets, fresh frozen plasma and cryoprecipitate (which contains fibrinogen, factor 8, Von Willibrand factor and factor).

When we say we are transfusing blood, we mean we are using packed red cells with no plasma, clotting factors, or other cells. The purpose is to increase oxygen carriage; there is no artificial substitute which will do this. We can use colloids to expand blood volume. In OMFS, we are likely to transfuse only if there has been significant blood loss, either as a result of major trauma or major surgery, usually a cancer resection.

Donated blood is processed into its constituents to use separately, so should a patient undergoing surgery be thrombocytopenic, we would request platelets. We would ask for fresh frozen plasma if the patient is bleeding and is short of clotting factors; most usually this would be if they have had massive bleeding and have been transfused a lot of red cells. There are boxes on the request form (or on screen) to ask for platelets or fresh frozen plasma. Always request a full blood count at the same time as you will need a baseline measurement of the haemoglobin.

The laboratory will test the sample for blood grouping using the ABO and Rhesus systems and then take donated red cells of the same compatible group and test them against serum from the patient's sample (cross match). In order to facilitate this, they will want to know if the blood group is already known and if the

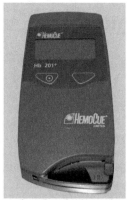

The HemoCue® haemoglobin analyser is kept in the operating theatre. It can produce a result within a few minutes on a blood sample taken from a thumb prick. The result is claimed to be as accurate as that from a venous sample assayed in the laboratory.

patient has had any previous transfusions or has been pregnant, as either of these may predispose to antibody formation.

If we know we will need blood in advance, for example, for planned major cancer surgery, we will tick the box on the request form for blood to be cross matched: we will say how many units we anticipate we will need and when we need it. Blood will then be cross matched and kept in the refrigerator to be collected. If we think we might need blood but are not definitely sure, then the lab will not want to cross match. In this case, you will tick the box to 'group and save'. This means the blood is tested for the group using ABO and Rhesus systems and the patient's serum is saved in the fridge to be used to cross match should they get a phone call from the operating theatre to say blood is needed.

You may find that the laboratory will prefer to receive a sample a week or so before to test for ABO and Rhesus grouping and to test for atypical antibodies, so that they are forewarned, and then another sample on the day of operation for cross matching.

You should know when a patient receives blood, it invariably leads to some pyrexia. Although the donated blood had been found to be compatible using the ABO and Rhesus systems and cross matched, there is always some degree of immunological reaction to it.

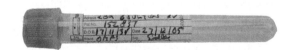

An EDTA containing tube is used for transfusion testing. Always hand write the details on the tube.

22. <u>Biopsy Techniques</u>

You will almost certainly will be taking biopsies of soft tissue lesions from within the mouth and will inevitably be asked to fill in request forms and label specimen bottles. You should attempt to get to know your friendly pathologist; he or she will almost certainly be keen to discuss specimens with you. Hopefully, there will be clinico-pathological conferences (CPCs) in your department where you can discuss clinical cases and look at the histopathology slides together. An understanding of pathology is essential to understanding disease; it will enrich your clinical learning and help with your postgraduate examinations.

When a lesion is removed entirely and sent for examination, the procedure is called an 'excisional biopsy' as opposed to an 'incisional biopsy' where a part of the lesion is removed. You should say on the request form which it is.

You should make your requests for histopathology with a clear, but not verbose, clinical history. These requests will mostly be made on the hospital's computer system via their Care Records System (CRS). Where they are still made on handwritten request forms, it will be appreciated if they are written legibly. You should include reference to any previous specimens and their laboratory numbers. Always make sure you have correctly labelled both the request form and the specimen bottle. For some oral lesions, such as suspected lichen planus, the history should include current drugs taken. For white patches, the pathologist should be told about smoking and drinking habits. We also encourage you to put down a short list of differential diagnoses.

The pathology report will include a macroscopic description of the specimen, a microscopic description of the material and a conclusion on the diagnosis; for a cancer resection, a comment will be made on the clearance at the margins of the lesion.

The pathological diagnosis may not be taken as gospel truth in every case. Sometimes a poor specimen has been provided, particularly one too small. Sometimes the specimen may be unrepresentative of the whole lesion. Remember that part of a white patch may show no dysplasia at all, whereas a few millimetres away a small invasive cancer may be developing. What is described as mildly, moderately or severely dysplastic will depend upon the individual pathologist's judgement and all of us are fallible.

Therefore, clinical decisions on management should not be based only on the histology report, although it will be very strong evidence. If a malignancy is suspected on clinical grounds but the histology fails to find any, the patient must not be dismissed but followed up and re-biopsy carried out if the lesion does not resolve quickly. Some pathological appearances, especially of bone, may represent a spectrum of abnormal activity such as fibrous dysplasia, ossifying fibroma and osteogenic sarcoma. Here, the pathologist may wish to see the X-rays or get the opinion of others. The bone tumour panel comprises a network of pathologists with a special interest in bony lesions; they will pass around borderline or other difficult specimens by post to provide supplementary opinions and reports.

In some cancer cases, specimens will be taken after the tumour has been resected to check that the margins have been cleared. The specimens will go straight to the laboratory where they will be frozen and stained before being examined by the pathologist who will give a verbal report to the surgeon in the operating theatre by telephone. This process is known as taking 'frozen sections'.

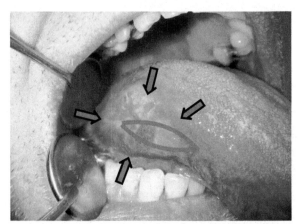

Incision margins for incisional biopsy of this obvious squamous cancer of the lateral margin of the tongue. The macroscopic margins of the tumour are marked with arrows

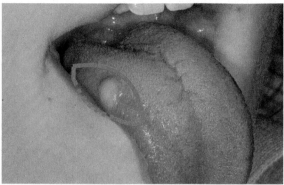

This lesion has all the clinical features of being benign so it is going to be removed completely. The incision margins for this excision biopsy are marked.

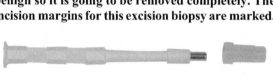

Disposable punch used for taking small biopsies. This is most useful for attached gingiva and for taking multiple samples from extensive white patches

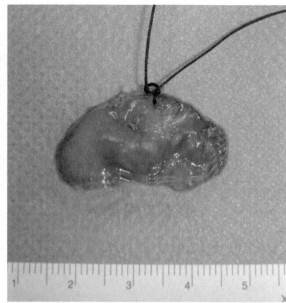

This specimen has been marked with a suture so the pathologist can orientate which way round it is.

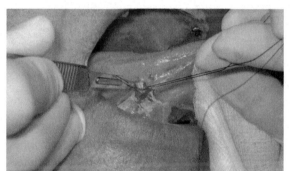

Any suspicious lesion should have a biopsy specimen taken for examination with a microscope. Here an incisional biopsy is is being taken. Part of the lesion, a floor of mouth keratosis, is being removed from the margin with some normal tissue.

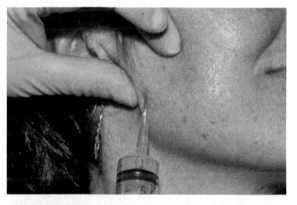

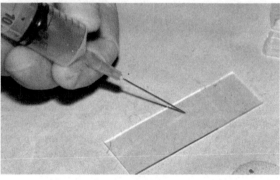

Fine needle aspiration cytology. A sample is taken from a parotid tumour (above) and gently put onto a slide to go to the laboratory.

Information needed with a histopathology request

- Patient's demographic details

- Specimen and request clearly labelled

- Brief description of lesion

- Brief history of complaint

- Smoking, drinking & medication if relevant

- Results of other investigations

- Provisional clinical diagnosis

The Laboratory Process

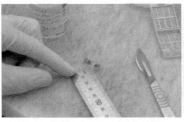
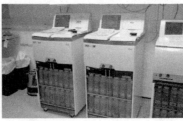
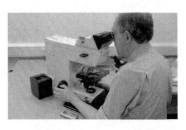

1. The process starts in the 'cut up' room. The pathologist is assisted by a secretary to whom he dictates his findings and measurements.

5. The machines remove all the moisture from the samples using various solvents.

8. The processed slides are presented to the pathologist who looks at them under the microscope and dictates his report. After typing by the secretary, a hard copy goes back to the pathologist who checks there are no mistakes; he then signs to 'authorise' it.

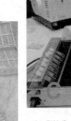

2. The specimen is described and measured for the macroscopic part of the report.

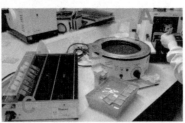

6. Slides are made from the wax blocks. The wax block is frozen, which facilitates easier cutting, and then sliced into thin layers with the microtome (A). A spatula is then used to transfer the wax sections into the water bath (B) where they float. A glass slide is then passed beneath the floating specimen and it is caught onto the slide which is then dried (C).

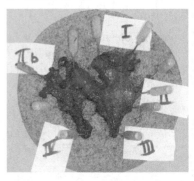

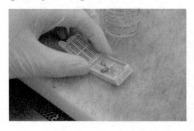

3. Pieces of the specimen are cut off and placed in a labelled cassette for processing into wax..

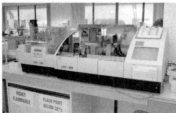

7. The slides then pass through the staining machine; this one is staining with haematoxylin and eosin.

Block dissection of lymph glands from the neck of a patient with intra oral carcinoma. The oncology team will want to know if any of the 40 plus glands in the specimen contain any cancer cells and if so whether there is any spread outside the capsule of the gland. This information is needed to stage the tumour and decide if post-operative radiotherapy is needed. The specimen has been pegged onto a cork board by the surgeon to help the pathologist orientate it and work out at what level in the neck he is taking glands from. A neck dissection will be time consuming work for the histopathologist. The levels of the neck 1, 2, 2b, 3 & 4 have been marked.

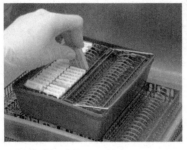

4. The cassette is placed, with others, in the rack for processing.

23. Cardiovascular and Respiratory Assessment

All patients coming into hospital for operation should have an assessment made of their cardiovascular and respiratory systems. Traditionally, the patient was "clerked" by a house officer on the ward. This involved a full history, examination and investigations such as blood tests, a chest radiograph and ECG. This has been superseded by dedicated nurse-led pre-operative assessment clinics.

Every patient receiving anaesthetic will be seen pre-operatively by an anaesthetist, who will go through their medical history and examine them as necessary. However, it is useful for OMFS trainees to appreciate systemic disease and how it may affect surgery and anaesthesia.

It should also be noted that as an OMFS trainee, you will assist in the management of post-operative patients on the ward. The post-operative period is critical; occasionally, these patients develop medical complications rather than complications from the actual surgery itself. In order to hand over to your senior colleagues, it will be helpful if you can understand what might happen and form a rough differential diagnosis.

The medical history is the most important part of eliciting disease; physical examination will usually only confirm what has already been suspected during history taking. A full medical clerking includes a history and examination of the cardiovascular, respiratory, gastrointestinal, renal, urinary, neurological and locomotor systems. We will address cardiovascular and respiratory health which will be most significant for most OMFS patients.

Recording of blood pressure is the first and probably the most important part of cardiovascular assessment. Hypertension is a risk factor for cardiovascular disease, especially heart failure, ischaemic heart disease, strokes and peripheral vascular disease as well as chronic kidney disease.

Update of important cardiac disease

A basic knowledge of common and serious cardiovascular and respiratory pathology will aid in putting clinical assessment and post-operative complications into context.

Heart failure is when the heart is having difficulty pumping blood (and therefore oxygen and nutrients) to the peripheral tissues. There are numerous causes of failure. Most commonly it will result from

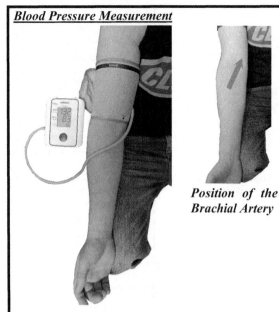

Blood Pressure Measurement

Position of the Brachial Artery

The sphygmomanometer cuff should fit snugly around the arm about 2cm above the ante-cubital space. Recline the patient comfortably. Palpate the brachial artery, then place the cuff with the arrow which is marked on the cuff approximating to the position of the artery. The cuff should be placed at the level of the heart. Palpate the radial pulse and inflate the cuff to 30 mm Hg above the level at which the radial pulse disappears.

A reading above 140/90 should be repeated. If this occurs over three occasions the GP should be informed so they can monitor and treat if necessary. If over 160/110 the anaesthetist may want to postpone a routine case until it is controlled. The risk of hypertension causing an adverse cardiovascular event during anaesthesia is not quantified, but should such an event occur no one would wish to feel responsible. It is important that all adults have their blood pressure measured intermittently. Hypertension is associated with a shortened life span due to its numerous complications. Atheroma formation is accelerated by hypertension so there is an increased risk of ischaemic heart disease, peripheral vascular disease, aneurysm and strokes. If severe it can cause myocardial hypertrophy and pulmonary venous congestion. It may affect the small vessels of the cerebral and renal circulation.

Symptom or Sign	Significance
Chest Pain	Angina:-cardiac muscle ischemia. Unusual as managed well medically or surgically esp. by angioplasty but may give a history
Shortness of breath (SOB)	Heart failure (left side) Unusual at rest as will be treated but may give a history. Ask about SOB on exertion
Orthopnoea	SOB on lying flat caused by heart failure. Ask if they need many pillows to sleep comfortably
Ankle swelling	Heart failure (right side). Will probably have been managed medically but may give a history
Faints or 'funny turns'	May be caused by arrhythmias. Should have an ECG to investigate
Palpations	May indicate arrhythmias, most commonly atrial fibrillation should have an ECG as it can easily lead to strokes
Claudication	Pain in calves on walking caused by peripheral vascular disease. May indicate widespread cardiovascular disease - myocardial ischemia risk of strokes and renal disease

Cardiovascular System Signs & Symptoms

myocardial ischaemia, hypertension, arrhythmias (often secondary to ischemia) or valve disease. Also metabolic diseases such as diabetes or thyroid disease, can cause failure, or any disease process which damages the cardiac muscle (myopathy). Sometimes failure may result from lung disease; chronic obstructive pulmonary disease (COPD) can cause pulmonary hypertension causing heart failure ("cor pulmonale").

The most common cause is ischaemic heart disease (IHD) where, through a lack of oxygen, the muscle of the myocardium has suffered irreversible damage and can no longer pump adequately. Most patients will give a history of angina, report a previous myocardial infarction or will have undergone angioplasty. Signs of IHD can also be found in some ECGs.Sometimes, the heart may fail because of a rhythm disorder (arrhythmias) secondary to IHD or old age; this is diagnosed by ECG. Atrial fibrillation (AF) is the most common rhythm abnormality causing heart failure. AF is diagnosed by feeling the peripheral pulse as "irregularly irregular". It is potentially dangerous as it leads to strokes and should be managed with anti-arrhythmics and anti-coagulants.

Valvular heart disease can cause heart failure when a valve is incompetent (incomplete closure of a valve causes retrograde flow) or stenosed (a stiff or thickened valve resists smooth anterograde flow). These may be suspected when an added heart sound or "murmur" may be heard on auscultation of the heart and confirmed by an ECHO cardiogram, a type of ultrasound examination.

In mild heart failure, the patient may have no symptoms at rest, but on exertion the diseased heart may not pump efficiently enough to provide adequate tissue oxygenation. This may cause shortness of breath on exertion.

The signs of failure can be understood by considering the two sides of the pumping heart.. The right side receives deoxygenated blood from the peripheral tissues and pumps this to the lungs. The left side receives oxygenated blood from the lungs and pumps this to the peripheral tissues. Blood restricted from efficient entry through a failing right side of the heart will lead to increased central venous pressure and fluid accumulation in the peripheries. This is seen clinically as a raised jugular venous pressure (JVP) and ankle, leg or sacral pitting oedema. Blood damming behind a failing left side of heart accumulates in the lungs, causing pulmonary oedema (producing shortness of breath) and in severe cases pleural effusions. This is detected clinically as basal crepitation on auscultation and dullness to percussion at the lung bases.

Respiratory disease

The most common respiratory disease you are likely to encounter is an upper respiratory tract infection (URTI). This is a relative contraindication to having general anaesthetic, as patients are more likely to get laryngo-bronchospasm with an endotracheal tube and there is an increased risk of pneumonia. Although it is sensible to delay surgery until at least two weeks after recovery, complications can, to a certain extent, be anticipated. Thus, it is prudent to continue with urgent surgery and delay only non-urgent cases.

Asthma is the most common co-existing chronic respiratory disease you are most likely to come across pre-operatively in young patients. Usually this is mild and patients will have the symptoms of wheezing or coughing only when they have a cold, and are controlled with a salbutamol +/- corticosteroid inhaler. These patients are managed easily by the anaesthetist.

Patients with more severe asthma may give a history of requiring previous hospital admissions or home nebuliser therapy. A nebuliser is a much more efficient and effective mechanism for delivering inhaled medication than inhalers. These patients may need a short course of steroids to prevent an acute attack and monitoring with a peak expiratory flow meter. Clinical signs on examination may include dyspnoea and wheeze during an attack, but otherwise would be expected to be normal.

Chronic obstructive pulmonary disease (COPD), unlike asthma, is largely irreversible airways constriction. It is commoner in older patients and is commonly associated with smoking. COPD patients exist on a spectrum where mild sufferers only develop shortness of breath on exertion, whereas in severe cases, patients require long-term oxygen therapy and nebulisers at home. Like asthmatics, they are likely to be on regular inhalers. Severe COPD patients will probably not be candidates for surgery under general anaesthetic unless for trauma or cancer. If you suspect that a patient is having an acute attack of asthma or COPD, seek help from medical colleagues as these patients may require oxygen, nebulisers and corticosteroids.

Some abnormal physical signs seen in respiratory disease are common to cardiovascular disease.

Symptom or Sign	Significance
Cough	Any cause of infection, inflammation or tumour. May be only symptom in asthma
Blood in sputum	May be caused by carcinoma but there are many other causes, should be thoroughly investigated
Shortness of Breath	Can be caused by most lung diseases particularly COPD and asthma as well as heart failure and anaemia
Wheeze	Commonly COPD & asthma but any cause of bronchial obstruction including tumour
Abnormal respiratory rate	Normally 12 - 16 per min. increased in any disease affecting respiratory exchange. Breathing out slowly through pursed lips occurs subconsciously to keep the airways open to the end of the respiratory cycle to aid gas exchange.

Respiratory System Signs & Symptoms

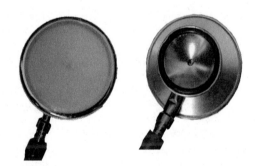

For examination both the bell and the diaphragm of the stethoscope should be used. The bell, pressed lightly on the chest wall, is best for hearing low pitched sounds, whereas the diaphragm is best used for high frequency sounds and is therefore used more frequently.

Examination

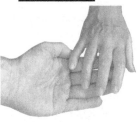

1. **Hands:** examine for nicotine staining, warmth and clubbing of the finger ends

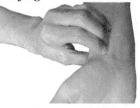

2. **Pulse:** two fingers are used to palpate the radial artery. Is the pulse 'full' or weak, regular or irregular? Count the pulse rate

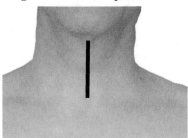

3. **Trachea:** Palpate: is it deviated to either side? Is there any deformity of the chest wall, do both sides expand equally during inspiration?

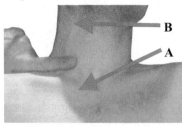

4. **Jugular Venous Pressure (JVP):** Recline the patient at 45° and ask them to look at a fixed point on their left. The JVP is normally 5 cms above the left atrium which is about 5cms below the manubrial sternal angle (arrow A). Put a finger across the external jugular at the base of the neck and press gently. A column of blood will become visible in the vein (arrow B), which will flow away when the finger is removed. In heart failure the column may be there without the external pressure. The JVP will be the height of any column of blood visible in the Internal Jugular Vein + 5 cms above the manubrial sternal angle (arrow A).

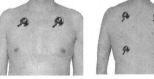

5. **Auscultate** the chest with the diaphragm of the stethoscope and percuss the upper lobes at the front and upper and lower lobes at the back. Examine beneath the axilla on the left for the middle lobe of the lung, there is no middle lobe on the right.

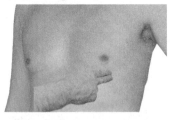

6. Palpate for the apex beat of the heart: it should normally be at the 5th intercostal space in the mid clavicular line. Also note whether there is a 'thrill' which is a palpable murmur and best felt with a flat palm held horizontally across the 2nd and 5th intercostal spaces in the mid clavicular line

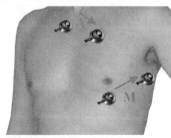

7. **Murmurs:** For mitral murmurs (Area M) listen at the 5th inter costal space (just beneath the left nipple) in the mid clavicle line. This is the mitral area (M) which extends from the apex to the mid axillary line. Mitral murmurs are often low pitched and 'rumbling'; best heard with the bell of the stethoscope. First listen with the patient sitting up, and holding his breath in full expiration. However, a quiet mitral murmur will best be heard with the patient lying on their left side in full expiration which brings the heart over towards the chest wall. While listening collate the findings with the cardiac cycle by palpating the carotid artery pulse. Aortic murmurs (Area A) tend to be more high pitched and are heard with the diaphragm of the stethoscope from the right of the sternum at the level of the first rib, passing over to the right of the sternum and down to the second intercostal space.

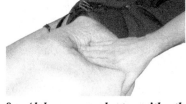

8. **Abdomen:** palpate with the patient lying flat with arms laid by his side. Palpate with the flat of the hand from the right iliac fossa to the right costal margin.

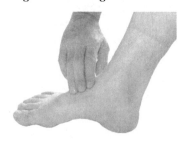

9. **Feet:** feel for the dorsalis pedis pulse which will be weak or absent in peripheral vascular disease. Examine for oedema consequent upon right sided heart failure. This will show 'pitting' if you push your thumb into it.

Notes on examination

1. Nicotine staining indicates smoking a risk factor for cardiovascular and respiratory disease. Severe pulmonary disease produces CO_2 retention, causing dilated peripheral veins and warm extremities. Very severe disease may produce peripheral cyanosis. 'Clubbing' of the finger over the distal phalanx may be congenital as in cyanotic heart disease or acquired as in endocarditis, chronic hypoxia, bronchogenic carcinoma, mesothelioma, interstitial lung disease, as well as certain gastrointestinal disease such as inflammatory bowel disease and liver disease. However, many cases are not associated with any underlying pathology.

2. The commonest irregularities are extra systoles which may occur regularly, or atrial fibrillation which always gives an irregular irregularity. These are indications for an ECG for more accurate diagnosis. Normal pulse rate is between 60 and 100 beats per minute with an average of 72 beats at rest. Even mild exercise or emotion will raise it. It will be higher in children, perhaps between 90 and 110, and lower in the elderly, 55 to 60. Well-trained athletes may have a low resting rate.

3. A trachea deviated from the midline is abnormal. The trachea may be deviated away from the side of a tension pneumothorax or large plural effusion or towards a lung which is collapsed, severely fibrosed or infiltrated with tumour. Movement of the chest wall may be reduced in certain pulmonary conditions, e.g. consolidation. Certain chest deformities, such as a barrel-shaped chest, suggest hyperinflation as may occur in COPD. Reduced lung expansion unilaterally may be due to lung collapse, pleural effusion or pneumothorax or bilateral in lung fibrosis.

4. The JVP is a rough approximation of the Central Venous Pressure (CVP) which will be increased in heart failure and decreased in hypovolaemia (significant blood loss). In a patient acutely ill with severe haemodynamic upset (or potentially so, such as in major surgery) this may be measured with a central CVP line and manometer. A specific measurement, as described, is probably too ambitious. It will usually be enough to say that the JVP is raised if the column of blood is anything other than not visible or just visible at the base of the neck.

5. For examination of the lung bases, the patient is asked to lean forward and cough. The base of the lung fields are auscultated for crepitations which sound like rustling tissue paper. Percussion of the basal lung fields may produce a dull note if there is a pleural effusion due to severe heart failure. A dull note will be heard in inflammation such as pneumonia. A hyper-resonant note may also be heard in pneumothorax or chronically where the lungs are hyper-inflated in COPD or asthma. Normal breath sounds are described as vesicular. A wheeze may be heard in asthma, and crackles may be heard in upper respiratory tract infection. Bronchial breathing is a harsh sound of air passing through the trachea and large airways. It may be heard over the peripheral lung fields if they are consolidated such as in pneumonia; this is because the sound will be conducted more efficiently.

6. Normally palpate with the flat of your hand to find the apex and then, when located, palpate more precisely with two fingers, as shown. The position of the apex beat may be displaced down and laterally if the left ventricle is hypertrophied, as may occur in valve disease or severe hypertension.

7. All diastolic murmurs are abnormal, but a systolic murmur may be an innocent 'flow' murmur if heard in very fit young adults or children; otherwise, systolic murmurs are usually due to aortic valve stenosis (common in the elderly) or mitral valve regurgitation. The finding of a murmur usually merits an ECHO cardiogram and a cardiologist's opinion.

8. An engorged liver from heart failure will be tender, smoothly enlarged, and palpable below the left costal margin. A normal liver should not be palpable. In severe heart failure, fluid may enter the peritoneal cavity (ascites). A large aortic aneurysm may be palpated by feeling centrally in the abdomen. It will expand in size with each heartbeat.

9. The dorsalis pedis pulse is felt in the first metatarsal space. Alternative is the posterior tibial artery midway between the medial malleolus (ankle) and the heel. In heart failure, fluid will accumulate in and around the systemic circulation. This will lead to an increased central venous pressure and hence JVP (see before), swelling of the feet or ankles and a smoothly enlarged tender liver. If the patient is bed bound, the fluid may accumulate in the sacral area rather than the feet. Atheromatous disease in the arteries may produce ischaemic heart disease, cerebrovascular accidents (strokes and transient ischaemic attacks), aneurysms and peripheral vascular disease. The latter may show as weak or absent pulses, cold feet, ulcers or gangrene.

24. Anaesthesia

The anaesthetist's role

As well as general anaesthesia anaesthetists also provide a sedation service, a pain relief service for obstetrics, run a chronic pain service for outpatients, supervise the nurse-provided acute pain service for inpatients, and they usually run the Intensive Care Unit. For OMFS anaesthetists do some sedation for patients with ischaemic heart disease or chronic obstructive pulmonary disease. For these patients, it is often safest to use local anaesthetic in the operating theatre with sedation, oxygen and monitoring provided by an anaesthetist. We may sedate patients having minor surgery ourselves with midazolam if they are medically fit, i.e. ASA grade 1 or 2.

During surgery, anaesthetists will be responsible for the patient's systemic well-being. They will normally visit the patient pre-operatively. They will administer the anaesthetic in the anaesthetic room, then transfer the patient to the theatre where they will monitor the anaesthetic and the patient's general condition.

In theatre, a trained anaesthetic nurse or an operating department practitioner (ODP) will assist the anaesthetist and draw up drugs and occasionally monitor the patient. In some hospitals, there are 'physician's assistants' who can give the whole anaesthetic supervised by an anaesthetist who might be elsewhere in the theatre suite.

The anaesthetist will expect to know exactly what the surgeon intends to do. They should be informed if anything out of the ordinary is contemplated, such as length of the surgery or special airway problems or requirements. Any pre-operative investigations needed should have been organised at a pre-admission clinic by nurses according to agreed protocols. All patients receiving a general anaesthetic for all but in 'emergency' operations should have been 'nil by mouth' according to local protocols. This ensures their stomachs are empty in order to minimise the risk of aspiration of stomach contents into the airway.

Securing the airway

For most OMFS surgery, anaesthetic gases will be delivered to the lungs via an endotracheal tube passed through the nose and known as a 'nasal tube'. This will be the most convenient for operating in the mouth as it will obviously not interfere with access to the operative site.

Sometimes, passing a tube through the nose may be difficult, such as in a patient with a deviated nasal septum or a history of trauma to the nose. Then it might be easier to work with an endotracheal tube passed through the mouth known as an 'oral tube'. It is quite usual to carry out many procedures in the mouth around an oral tube, particularly unilateral ones, although it requires some adaption by the surgeon. Some procedures are not possible with an oral tube, such as reduction and fixation of fractures where you will need to occlude the teeth together during the operation. A third possibility is a laryngeal mask. Here the anaesthetic gas is passed through a rather thicker tube and the seal with the airway is made at the larynx by contact with a fairly bulky mask apparatus. From the anaesthetic point of view, it does away with the need to pass a tube through the larynx into the trachea so the patient does not require paralysing and the anaesthetic process is much quicker. The tube is quite bulky and can be difficult to work round and, if you are not used to working with a laryngeal mask, it is quite possible that you may dislodge it during the procedure. However, an experienced surgeon can frequently work adequately

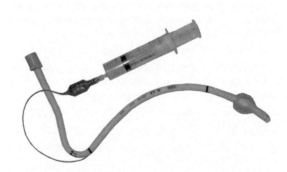

The endotrachael tube prepared for the anaesthetist by the ODP. It has a cuff which is inflated with air from a syringe to make a seal within the trachea

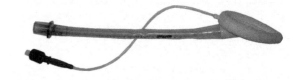

Laryngeal mask airway (LMA)

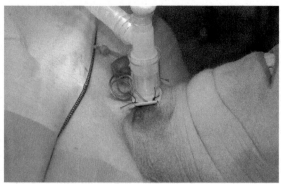

Anaesthetic breathing circuit attached to a tracheostomy tube for a major cancer case

around a laryngeal mask, which has been expertly placed.

Sometimes an anaesthetic is delivered through a tracheostomy. This is reserved for our major head and neck cancer patients and those with severe facial trauma. The patient is anaesthetised in the conventional manner and an oral tube placed, then a tracheostomy is made and a tube passed into the trachea as the anaesthetist withdraws the oral tube. Now the surgeon can operate anywhere in the head and neck without compromising the airway and is secure knowing that the airway will not be affected by post-operative swelling or bleeding.

The anaesthetist will normally place a pack in the pharynx at the beginning of the surgery to catch blood or other debris. The pack remains the responsibility of the anaesthetist and at the end of the operation, the surgeon should ask the anaesthetist if he wants the pack removed. When confirmed, it should be removed, and the pharynx sucked out. This should include careful suction of the postnasal space under direct vision or blood clots caused by bleeding during nasal intubation. The anaesthetist will normally check the pharynx themselves using a laryngoscope before they wake the patient up.

The anaesthetic room process

Once in the anaesthetic room, the anaesthetist will again check the patient's wristband and ask the patient to confirm their identity. The anaesthetic can then commence. The first task is to place an IV cannula, the ODP will have drawn up all the drugs needed into syringes and labelled them. The anaesthetic is usually induced with an intravenous infusion of an anaesthetic drug such as propofol. Sometimes the patient may be induced by breathing an inhalation anaesthetic through a mask. Once consciousness is lost, the patient will be ventilated with a face mask using an inhalation

anaesthetic carried in a mixture of nitrous oxide and oxygen. Once they are deep enough, a muscle relaxant is given, and a tube passed. The tube is then connected to the anaesthetic machine via a 'breathing circuit' and secured. The patient's eyes are covered to prevent accidental injury.

Once the patient is anaesthetised, there are other preparations to make before they are ready for surgery. For major cases, this may include an arterial line to measure blood pressure directly and to sample for blood gases and pH levels. A central venous pressure line will help gauge fluid status and a cerebral function monitor will measure the depth of the anaesthetic. Once the anaesthetic has been administered, the patient will be transferred to the operating theatre where they will be connected to a blood pressure cuff and a pulse oximeter. There may be a urinary catheter to monitor urine output and a temperature probe (often in the urinary catheter) to measure core body temperature. A naso-gastric tube may be passed to aspirate stomach secretions and prevent regurgitation. The patient may be covered in an inflatable blanket to maintain their temperature and have pneumatic compression stockings to gently squeeze their calves. This is to prevent thrombosis in the large veins in the legs, which can be fatal if a clot should embolise and pass into the lungs.

A more recent development is the Total Intravenous Anaesthetic (TIVA). Here, the propofol used for induction is continued, using a syringe driver throughout the operation. This may be accompanied by a continuous infusion of a short-acting opiate such as remifentanil. In this technique, the only gas delivered to the patient's lungs is a mixture of oxygen and air.

During surgery, the anaesthetist and ODP will monitor the patient and record the progress on the anaesthetic chart. They will administer any drugs and at the end will wake the patient up and accompany them to the recovery room, handing their care over to the recovery nurse. The patient remains the anaesthetist's responsibility while they are still in the theatre suite. The recovery nurse will ask the anaesthetist's permission to send the patient back to the ward when they have recovered sufficiently.

The anaesthetist will ensure that the patient has post-operative analgesia prescribed for the post-operative period. They regard this as one of their responsibilities and are normally very keen that we inject a long-acting local anaesthetic with a vasoconstrictor around the operation site as it contributes to a more comfortable recovery.

The anaesthetic process

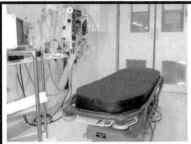

1. The patient is brought to the anaesthetic room will have all the anaesthetic equipment of the theatre itself

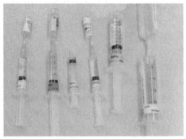

Drugs will have been drawn up and labelled by the anaesthetic nurse or ODP. From left: Dexamethasone (steroid to reduce swelling & anti-emetic), Mivacurium (short acting non depolarising muscle relaxant), Atropine (antimuscarinic), Ondansetron (anti-emetic), Morphine (opiate analgesic), Co-amoxiclav (antibiotic)

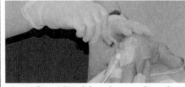

2. After the identity and safety checks a cannula is placed and anaesthesia is usually induced

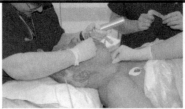

3. Once the patient has been induced IV an endotracheal tube is place. Here an oral tube is being passing though the vocal cords into the trachea with direct vision using the laryngoscope. This is helped by an assistant putting downward pressure on

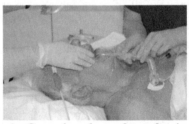

4. Once in place the tube is connected to the anaesthetic circuit and secured. The position is checked by inflating the lungs by squeezing the gas reservoir bag and listening to the chest with a stethoscope. The correct position will also be confirmed by looking at the observation monitor which will show the presence of expired CO_2. The eyes are taped shut and protected

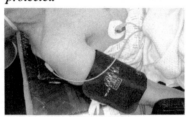
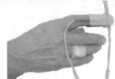

5. ECG leads, a blood pressure cuff and a pulse oximeter are attached to the patient

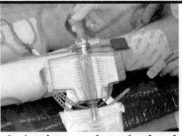

6. A urinary catheter is placed so that fluid output can be measured, the catheter contains a temperature probe to measure core body temperature

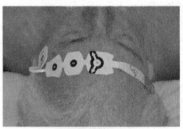
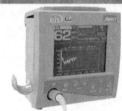

Bispectral index cerebral function monitor. It monitors the depth of anaesthesia by recording electrical activity (Electroencephalography or EEG)

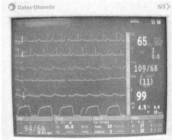

The video monitor during a major case. It shows ECG, pulse rate, blood pressure, O2 saturation, expired CO2, central venous pressure, direct arterial pressure & temperature

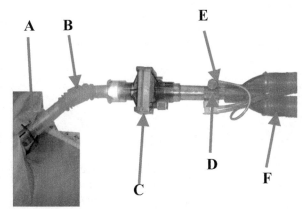

Breathing circuit: A: *Endotrachael tube passing into patient's mouth* **B**: *Connector to tube* **C**: *Gas filter/humidifier* **D**: *Gas pressure/flow monitor* **E**: *Gas (O₂, N₂O and anaesthetic vapour monitor system* **F**: *Anaesthetic gases circuit, in and out*

We have already mentioned that in much OMFS we are attempting to share the upper airway with the anaesthetist. This can cause potential difficulties. In addition, there will be several specific problems related to our patients which might cause difficulty with conventional intubation. The anaesthetist will want to be forewarned of these so that he can modify his technique. These include patients with obstruction to the airway as a result of cancer or trauma, abnormality of anatomy such as severe retrognathia, limitation of jaw opening consequent upon jaw ankylosis, and fractures of the mandible, maxilla or malar. A common problem is limited mouth opening caused by an acute dental abscess.

The anaesthetist will always assess the difficulty or ease of intubation before starting. This assessment will involve an examination of the patient's neck. Difficulty can be anticipated in patients with short, fat necks and those with reduced neck flexion as might be caused by arthritis. They will assess jaw movement in an anterior posterior direction, but most particularly mouth opening. They may do this using the Mallampati test, which is a grading of visibility of mouth structures with the patient sitting in a head neutral position; the patient is asked to open their mouth as wide as possible and fully protrude their tongue. If this gives full visibility of the tonsils, uvula and soft palate, this is a good sign, but if only the hard palate can be seen, this is a sign that conventional intubation might be difficult.

If a patient is given a conventional anaesthetic induction with propofol and a muscle relaxant and then the anaesthetist cannot place a tube in the trachea, this is potentially dangerous as the airway might be lost.

An alternative technique is to give the patient a gas induction so that he breathes into a deep anaesthetic without a muscle relaxant. However, this might be problematical if it is difficult to get a good air seal with a face mask because of abnormal anatomy, facial trauma or a beard, or if the patient is obese. They might de-saturate their oxygen concentration quickly. For potentially difficult intubation cases, the anaesthetist may use a video laryngoscope to get an improved view of the glottis to facilitate a safer intubation of a fibre-optic intubation technique.

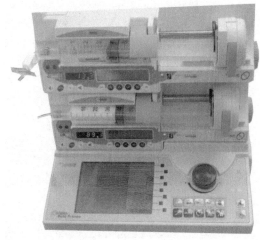

TIVA. Propofol and Remifentanil being administered by continuous infusion from a syringe driver

Anaesthetic machine

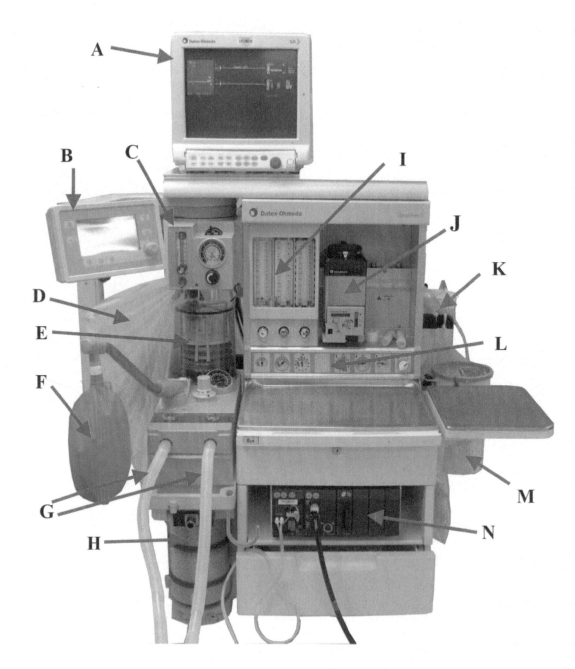

A: *Monitor* B: *Ventilator control system* C: *Suction control* D: *Clinical waste bag* E: *Ventilator bellows* F: *Reservoir bag* G: *Anaesthetic gas circuit, in and out* H: *CO_2 scavenger* I: *Gases flow meters* J: *Vaporiser for anaesthetic* K: *Suction chamber* L: *Gas pressure gauges* M: *Sharps box* N: *Monitoring modules for blood pressure, O_2 saturation, arterial pressure, central venous pressure, temperature*

25. <u>Sedation</u>

For the vast majority of patients receiving dental treatment, local anaesthesia will be used alone. However, many patients will be anxious and as minor oral surgery may be justifiably viewed as particularly unpleasant, they may request a general anaesthetic. Many prospective patients will be ignorant of the potential risks of general anaesthesia. The additional costs involved in making it safe will frequently lead to delays in them receiving the requested treatment.

In most cases, conscious sedation will be an acceptable alternative and can be administered safely by the surgeon in a dental facility. However, the availability in OMFS departments may sometimes be limited by a policy of it only being provided in an operating theatre by an anaesthetist; this reduces the cost advantage.

Sedation is defined as:

a technique in which the use of a drug or drugs produces a state of depression of the central nervous system, enabling treatment to be carried out, but during which verbal contact with the patient is maintained throughout the period of sedation.

The technique used to provide conscious sedation for dental treatment should carry a margin of safety wide enough to render a loss of consciousness unlikely. This is usually easily accomplished with intra-venous midazolam.

Consent for treatment should preferably be obtained on a day prior to the actual treatment when the patient is assessed for their oral and general medical state. This should be confirmed on the day of treatment. The patient should be given written information about sedation. If the patient is in pain and immediate treatment needed, this ideal will not be possible. Adult patients receiving the usual moderate sedation for treatment will maintain their normal reflexes and swallowing ability, so should not need to starve beforehand. However, children should have no fluids for two hours beforehand and no solids for six.

Assessment for sedation should include a full medical and dental history and baseline vital signs should be recorded including blood pressure, pulse and respiratory rates and oxygen saturation. Patients for outpatient surgery with sedation administered by a dental operator/sedationist should be ASA grading 1 or 2 (see Chapter 4 for ASA grading). They should be given verbal and written instructions which should include the advice not to have alcohol or recreational

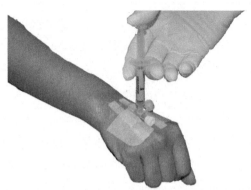

Sedation for minor oral surgery is usually Midazolam administered through a 22G or 24G cannula

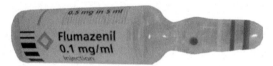

Flumazenil should be available to reverse the midazolam in the rare occasion when the patient has become over sedated

drugs for 24 hours beforehand. They should be accompanied by a responsible adult.

Inhalation sedation using nitrous oxide and oxygen may be used for minor oral surgery or oral sedation using temazepam or midazolam. However, mostly because of variation in individual response, this is less predictable than intravenous midazolam, which is the most common technique for oral surgery.

Midazolam produces anxiolysis and sedation; it produces amnesia and has a high therapeutic index so that there is a wide margin between adequate sedation and loss of consciousness. It is, therefore, safe and can be given by the operator. Oral surgery can be unpleasant, so the amnesia is welcome.

In some situations, midazolam may be combined with the opiate fentanyl or the anaesthetic agent propofol. These techniques are unsuitable for use by an operator/sedationist in the dental surgery because it is less easy to titrate the doses. Also there will be a lower margin between moderate sedation and the patient becoming unconscious. These techniques are used by anaesthetists in the operating theatre.

Whilst it is permissible for the operator to give the sedation, they should have received training and be accompanied by two nurses who have received training. Dental nurses can take the National

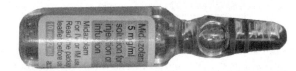

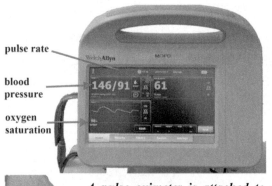

pulse rate

blood
pressure

oxygen
saturation

146/91   61

A pulse oximeter is attached to a finger and used to monitor the oxygen saturation throughout the procedure. Oxygen saturation, pulse rate, respiratory rate and blood pressure should be recorded every 5 minutes.

Midazolam

Is a benzodiazepine

Is quick to act

Half life for elimination is 3 to 4 hours

Has a wide margin of safety

Is sedative

Is anxiolytic

Produces amnesia

Examining Board for Dental Nurses' certificate in Dental Sedation Nursing. One nurse should assist in the surgery and one should monitor the patient's vital signs and record them every 5 minutes. There should be appropriate recovery facilities. Afterwards, the patient should remain at least an hour after the last dose of midazolam and until they can walk unaided and talk coherently. They should be accompanied home by a responsible adult.

The midazolam is given through an intravenous cannula and titrated in slowly. Initially, 2 mg are slowly injected over 30 seconds and then after a pause of at least a minute, further increments of 1 mg can be given until the patient is relaxed enough for treatment to start; the dose required normally varies between 2 and 7.5 mg. The signs of adequate sedation include the patient being relaxed, slurred speech and partial ptosis. They should always be able to maintain verbal contact.

Using this technique, most patients who are excessively apprehensive about minor oral surgery and who are demanding a general anaesthetic can be persuaded to have sedation instead. The amnesic effect of midazolam is remarkable so that most have no recollection of the surgery at all.

It is essential that the surgeon should not be left alone with a sedated patient. Not only is it possible that they may need help in the unlikely event that there is a medical emergency, but benzodiazepines have been associated with erotic dreams. There have been a few occasions in the past where patients have complained they have been interfered with.

Oral and maxillofacial departments receive a number of referrals from primary care dentists requesting extractions or minor oral surgery who are medically unwell. In many cases, particularly where there is severe cardiac or respiratory disease, these patients may be best served by having the surgery carried out with monitoring by an anaesthetist. Anaesthetists generally work in operating theatres where these patients may get continuous oxygen through a nasal cannula and monitoring with ECG, blood pressure and pulse oximetry. The anaesthetist may use advanced conscious sedation, usually with midazolam combined with propofol or fentanyl (opiate).

26. <u>Radiotherapy and its Oral Complications</u>

Mechanism of action.

Oral cancer is primarily squamous cell which is sensitive to radiotherapy. Radiotherapy uses high energy ionising radiation to generate free radicals which break double-stranded DNA, thus damaging the reproductive activity of cells leading to their death when they attempt to divide at mitosis. The dead cells are then removed by the body's own defence mechanism. Normal cells are damaged in the same way as malignant cells, but unlike the cancer cells, they can repair; they are thus much less affected.

Indications for radiotherapy.

Mouth cancer is usually treated primarily by surgery with radiotherapy used as an adjunct, normally afterwards. The blood supply of the normal tissues is adversely affected by radiotherapy and thus reduces their ability to heal, which is why surgery is usually done first. Early cancers are often treated with surgery alone. The indications for radiotherapy include positive lymph nodes in the neck, particularly multiple nodes or spread outside the capsule of the glands, and close surgical margins or poor differentiation of the tumour, as seen in the histology of the surgical specimens.

Oro-pharyngeal cancer (base of tongue, tonsil and pharynx) related to Human Papilloma Virus mostly occurs in younger patients who tend to be to otherwise healthier with their condition unrelated to smoking and high alcohol. These cases usually have a better prognosis and are often treated using chemotherapy and radiotherapy without surgery.

Radiotherapy can be used as part of attempted 'curative' treatment to destroy the tumour or reduce the chance of it recurring after surgery or as part of 'palliative' treatment where the chance of a cure has passed and the clinician has the more limited expectation of shrinking the tumour or alleviating pain.

Delivery of radiotherapy.

Head and neck tumours are treated with external beam radiotherapy delivered by a linear accelerator. Radiotherapy doses are expressed in Grays (Gy); a Gray is the radiation dose producing one joule of energy absorbed per kilogram of tissue. The dose is normally given divided into daily 'fractions' with time between, which allows the normal tissues to recover; this helps maintain oxygenation of the tumour, hypoxic tissues being less sensitive to radiation. Once a radiotherapy regime has started, it should not be

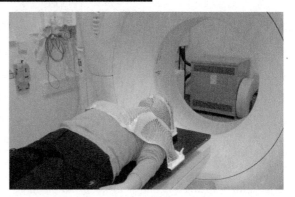

The patient is wearing a bespoke immobilization mask made of a thermoplastic material to hold her head in a reproducible position for a pre-treatment CT scan for radiotherapy planning.

Radiotherapy terminology

Curative: to cure the cancer
Adjuvant: after surgery to prevent recurrence
Neoadjuvant: to reduce the size of the tumour
prior to surgery
Palliative: to decrease severity and delay
progression

---

interrupted. Delay in starting the radiotherapy is undesirable, but it is not as detrimental to the outcome as interruption once treatment has started.

Intensity Modulated Radio Therapy (IMRT) involves many hundreds of small beams of radiation delivered to the tumour precisely, with sparing of the normal tissues. It is particularly used for head and neck cancer treatment because there are many structures which will benefit from avoiding radiation, such as the salivary glands, spinal cord and larynx. IMRT has been proved to reduce less long-term side effects, particularly the salivary glands reducing xerostomia; radical IMRT is the standard of care that should be provided for head and neck cancer patients.

Planning radiotherapy.

The planning process for radiotherapy treatment involves a CT scan taken with the patient wearing an immobilisation shell; the radiotherapist will then outline the tumour and sensitive structures, e.g. spinal cord and salivary glands on the scan. An MRI scan can be overlaid onto the CT image on the computer to give more information, but the actual doses will be calculated by the computer based on the density of the tumour, which is informed by the CT scan. The

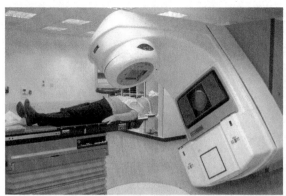

Patient receiving radiotherapy from linear accelerator wearing the mask to keep her head in reproducible position. (Simulated, not a real patient)

radiotherapist then checks with the MRI scan that all the tumour has been included in the radiation fields. Three-dimensional images can be very helpful in the planning. When the radiotherapist has prescribed the dose of radiation, marked out the volume to be treated and the structures to be avoided, a technologist plans the treatment on the computer.

Side effects.

The most immediate side effect of radiotherapy on the head and neck is mucositis, which usually manifests by the second or third week of treatment. It consists of widespread erythema, ulceration bleeding and pain. The oral and pharyngeal mucosa will become inflamed and possibly ulcerated. Maintenance of oral hygiene will be difficult when the mouth is so sore and this may be helped by chlorhexidine mouthwash to help with plaque control. The discomfort will significantly affect the ability to chew and swallow and hence impede nutrition. This may to some extent be helped by using a high calorie liquid diet and topical analgesic mouthwash, gargle, or spray (benzydamine hydrochloride).

In many cases, particularly where radiotherapy is combined with chemotherapy, feeding is delivered through a gastrostomy tube placed before treatment starts. A fine bore tube is inserted through the skin directly into the stomach, usually guided into the correct place with the aid of X-rays or ultrasound. Pain should be treated, and the patient encouraged to swallow something rather than rely entirely on the gastrostomy tube. The cells of the mucosa exhibit a high rate of turnover, so the mucositis can be expected to recover about three weeks after completion of treatment.

Oral side effects of Radiotherapy

1. Mucositis

Soreness

Ulceration

Bleeding

Difficulty eating

Difficult swallowing

Difficult oral hygiene

2. Xerostomia

Discomfort

Difficulty eating

Difficult swallowing

Increased periodontal disease

Increased caries

Secondary infection particularly candidiasis

3. Decreased vascularity of soft tissues

Poor healing, particularly after further surgery

Skin pigmentation

4. Fibrosis

Trismus

Difficulty eating

Difficult oral hygiene

Difficult dental treatment

Radiotherapy will have a permanent effect on the salivary glands, both major and minor, causing permanent damage and dryness of the mouth with such saliva as there is being thick. Whereas the effect is likely to be less with Intensity Modulated Radiotherapy, the xerostomia caused will be permanent.

There are a variety of different saliva substitutes available to help with symptoms, but our experience has been that patients often feel more comfortable carrying a bottle of water to use for symptomatic relief. Eventually patients seem to accommodate to the permanent dryness of the mouth with modulation of their diet, but the xerostomia has a permanent effect on their dental health because of the decreased salivary buffering and a higher rate of caries will ensue; this may be helped with fluoride mouth rinses.

In the short term, the mouth may be affected by secondary infection, particularly candidiasis, mucositis and ulceration. This may be helped by meticulous oral hygiene and antifungals, such as miconazole or fluconazole. Herpes simplex may be reactivated which can be helped with acyclovir.

Radiotherapy will permanently decrease the blood supply in the soft tissues it passes through. This will severely decrease the ability of these tissues to heal should they suffer any trauma or further surgery.

Complications: osteoradionecrosis.

Radiation obliterates blood vessels supplying the bone, as well as the soft tissues, so that it is deprived of nutriments and oxygen. This severely curtails its capacity to remodel, resist infection, and heal after trauma. This produces the most serious complication of head and neck radiotherapy, osteoradionecrosis. It mainly affects the mandible and is defined as irradiated bone which has undergone necrosis and remains exposed through the overlying soft tissues for over 3 months..

Necrotic bone may not be a problem for the patient until it becomes infected (particularly from periodontal or apical dental infection) or traumatised (particularly by dental extraction). Once infected, the necrotic bone will drain pus into the mouth, become permanently exposed to the mouth, and never heal. Risk factors are higher radiotherapy doses, smoking, high alcohol intake, periodontal disease and poor oral hygiene.

There will be permanent discharge with discomfort and unpleasant smell. There are likely to be acute exacerbations of the chronic infection with swelling and pain and a risk of pathological fracture. Where there are only small spicules of bone being discharged, healing may occur.

Osteoradionecrosis may be treated with PENTOCLO (Pentoxifylline, Tocopherol and Clodronate) but this requires further trials before it can be proved as effective. Hyperbaric oxygen has been used in the past but has now been mostly discontinued. Where necrosis is established, there is a choice between leaving it and accepting the discomfort and disability or surgery. It can lead to chronic extra oral fistulae or

Osteoradionecrosis risk factors
High dose of radiation
Alcohol
Smoking
Periodontal disease
Dental caries
Poor oral hygiene

Complications of Oral Radiotherapy
1. Osteoradionecrosis
Discharge
Bad smell & taste
Episodes of acute inflammation and pain
Fistulae
Pathological fracture
2. New tumours
Particularly in children
3. Compromised growth
In children

pathological fracture, so major surgery may be undertaken to remove all the necrotic bone and reconstruct with free vascularised bone grafts. Many of the patients will be elderly and frail and may not wish to have more major surgery after their cancer treatment. The damage to bone from radiotherapy is permanent, so patients are at risk of septic osteoradionecrosis from dental infection or extraction for the rest of their lives.

Radiotherapy will reduce vascularity to the soft tissues. This will cause reduced healing, which is why we prefer to carry out surgery prior to radiotherapy. The skin may become pigmented and the soft tissues will also be prone to fibrosis which may be responsible for limitation of mouth opening, particularly if the medial pterygoid and masseter muscles are included in high dose volume of treatment.

In the long term, radiotherapy increases the risk of the development of new tumours in the irradiated tissues. This has most significance in children who have received radiation for rare childhood tumours. It will also have a detrimental effect on growth in these children. Although IMRT reduces the short term side effects of radiotherapy, it involves more of the normal tissues receiving radiation.

Dental Management.

It is essential that all patients with oral, nasal or pharyngeal tumours should have a comprehensive assessment of their dentition as soon as they are diagnosed so that they are rendered dentally fit before treatment starts. In most centres, the patients are assessed by a restorative dentist, which will give the patient the opportunity to discuss future prosthetic rehabilitation. Any dental treatment or assessment should not be allowed to delay cancer treatment.

We tend to take a pessimistic approach to future dental health and plan treatment accordingly. In assessing the dentition, we acknowledge that most of the patients will be elderly and may have less than ideal periodontal conditions. Radiotherapy will cause xerostomia, leading to increased caries risk and that radiotherapy and surgery may lead to some degree of trismus, making oral hygiene measures and dental inspection or treatment difficult. This and the experience that osteoradionecrosis is so miserable for the patient usually means we recommend a radical approach and that any teeth which are not completely healthy in terms of tooth substance and periodontium which are in the field of high dose radiation are removed before treatment.

Where patients present and need dental extractions in areas of previous radiotherapy, if the extractions are essential, then they are usually given chlorhexidine mouthwashes and antibiotics. Pre extraction hyperbaric oxygen has not been shown to be effective. Otherwise patients who have had radiotherapy should have regular dental assessments, meticulous oral hygiene management and fluoride mouthwashes.

Which Scan?

Computerized tomography (CT)

Most cases will have a CT scan. As it is based on X-rays it shows bone best. Radiotherapy is planned on a CT scan. Usually the scan is made after the patient is injected with a contrast medium to improve the image of the tumour. A CT of the chest is used to show up any metastatic tumour.

Magnetic Resonance Imaging (MRI)

Many cases of oral cancer can barely be seen on CT because the density of the tumour may be very close to that of the normal tissue. MRI will show up a huge signal variation so that soft tissue tumours can be seen clearly. Sometimes a CT is poor due to artefacts cause by dental fillings. All patients should therefore ideally have both scans especially for oral cancers.

Positron Emission Tomography (PET)

Is used when we don't know where the primary is. Sometimes a patient presents with metastatic nodes in the neck. If pan-endoscopy of the upper aero-digestive tract does not reveal the primary a PET scan may show up a suspicious area to be biopsied carefully.

PET scan shows inflammation so biopsies should be done after the scan as it might be difficult the differentiate inflammation from cancer. Often it will show up a tumour in the tongue base (with overlying mucosa looking intact) or in the pyriform fossa or tonsillar region that you haven't been able to get access to examine properly.

PET scans are useful for post treatment assessment in some cases particularly patients who have had chemo-radiotherapy for metastatic disease. A PET scan at three months post-treatment may show up residual disease which would indicate that neck dissection is required.

27. Chemotherapy and its Oral Complications

Use of chemotherapy

Chemotherapy is the use of anti-cancer drugs to treat a wide variety of malignant conditions, particularly haemopoietic diseases such as leukaemias and lymphomas. It is also used against malignant cells metastasising from solid tumours such as breast and bowel cancer. The agents used are usually given in combinations and at high dose to target actively dividing cancer cells. However, they also have a wide range of nonspecific actions, which will have an adverse effect on normal tissues, particularly those with a high rate of cell turnover. Thus, the bone marrow, mucosa and salivary glands will be affected, which will be detrimental to oral health and need consideration when patients need oral or dental surgery.

When used in the management of head and neck, cancer chemotherapy is usually administered concomitantly with radiotherapy (chemoradiotherapy), usually for treatment of the more advanced cancers. For head and neck cancer, cisplatin is used as a radiosensitizer together with cetuximab, an epidermal growth factor receptor blocker. This also acts as a radiosensitizer, but with different toxicities to cisplatin. Chemotherapy is only rarely used for head and neck cancer without radiotherapy; this may be for palliation when the chance of a cure has passed or occasionally used before radiotherapy to shrink the tumour down before radiotherapy starts.

Side effects

Chemotherapy may cause mucositis, leading to ulceration and discomfort with resulting difficulty in chewing and swallowing. Mucositis will be temporary and may be helped by mouthwashes such as benzydamine hydrochloride or ice. There will be taste dysfunction which will exacerbate the chewing and swallowing problems caused primarily by the mucositis; salivary gland function may be impaired by anti-cholinergic medication given as an adjunct to the chemotherapy.

The most significant effect of chemotherapy affecting dental care will be myelosuppression (bone marrow suppression) causing leucopenia and thrombocytopenia. The reduced white cell count will lead to immunosuppression and, together with a reduction in saliva production, will frequently lead to candidiasis, which will further exacerbate the discomfort and dysphagia. Patients who are expected to be neutropenic because of chemotherapy are usually treated prophylactically with fluconazole; IV amphotericin may also be used.

Myelosuppression can be expected to be most problematical in patients receiving chemotherapy for leukaemias and lymphomas, and most particularly those receiving stem cell transplants. Suppression will be significant for about six weeks after chemotherapy has finished. During this time, the patient will be susceptible to becoming significantly unwell from dental infection or from other sources. An acute dental infection in a neutropenic patient may produce little or no pus, as there are few neutrophils from which pus can be formed. There may, therefore, be little or no pain but still cause the patient to be systemically unwell. A patient presenting with pyrexia during or soon after chemotherapy should be treated as an acute medical emergency by the oncology team according to the hospital's 'neutropenic sepsis' policy. They may be referred for a dental assessment as a tooth may be the cause.

Considerations before surgery

Patients who are expected to become neutropenic from chemotherapy should ideally have their dentition optimised beforehand, if time allows. An asymptomatic tooth with a chronic apical infection which has been draining, or a non-vital tooth with an apical radiolucency with no discharge may become dangerous during neutropenia. Then the balance of resistance will favour sepsis, pre-treatment extraction is to be preferred.

Thrombocytopenia during or after chemotherapy may lead to bleeding from periodontal inflammation and prolonged bleeding following dental extraction. However, we have far more platelets than are needed and the platelet count can be reduced considerably before bleeding becomes a practical problem. If an extraction is contemplated, a haematologist should be consulted if the count is less than 50×10^9 per litre as they may prescribe a platelet transfusion. If the extraction is not urgent, you can wait until it returns to above 100×10^9 per litre when the marrow is recovering from the chemotherapy.

Most of the side effects of chemotherapy on the mouth are temporary and will be expected to resolve with time.

28. <u>Anticoagulants and Surgery</u>

Uses of anticoagulation

Many patients are receiving anticoagulant therapy because they are at risk of thromboembolism because of atrial fibrillation, previous thrombosis or because they have mechanical heart valves. Most of them will receive the coumarin drug warfarin, which works by blocking the formation of prothrombin and clotting factors 2, 7, 9 and 10. It prevents the metabolism of vitamin K to its active form for synthesis of these factors. Warfarin binds strongly to plasma proteins so it has a long half-life of about 36 hours. This means the full anticoagulant effects take some time to be reached and continue for several days after the medication is stopped.

International Normalised Ratio

Anticoagulation is measured with the prothrombin test and is expressed as the INR (International Normalised Ratio) which is the ratio of the prothrombin time divided by a laboratory control. An INR of 1 would be normal, i.e. no anticoagulation, and 2 would mean the blood would take twice as long to clot. Patients have their warfarin doses adjusted to achieve the INR appropriate to the problem they have, which might lead to thromboembolism. This will be between 2 and 3 for patients at risk because of atrial fibrillation, a previous deep vein thrombosis or pulmonary embolism or transient ischemic events or strokes. A higher ratio of between 3 and 4 is appropriate for those who are at risk because of heart valve disorders, including mechanical heart valves or a recent myocardial infarct.

Management of patients on warfarin

It has been shown that patients who are anticoagulated within these therapeutic ranges of INR 2-4 are likely to have some additional risk of bleeding if they have minor oral surgery, including dental extractions. However, when they bleed, this can usually be stopped by simple local measures such as packing, suturing and tranexamic acid used locally. Stopping the anticoagulation places them at increased risk of rebound thrombosis, so it is recommended that no adjustment is appropriate if the patient's INR is within the therapeutic range (INR <4).

Patients who take warfarin will have an anticoagulant card with all their blood results on it. If they have a stable result, they should not need to come to hospital for dental extractions. However, some patients will have confounding factors, which put them at additional risk. These include unstable and variable INR, additional disease processes which might affect their coagulation, such as liver disease, renal failure, other coagulopathy or history of alcohol abuse. Some patients may take additional medication which may potentiate warfarin, such as anti-hypertensives, antifungals, carbamazepine, steroids, phenytoin, aspirin, and antibiotics such as erythromycin and metronidazole. In these situations, treatment in hospital will give the patient greater confidence that should excess bleeding occur, measures will be quickly available to help.

In all cases, oral wounds should be packed with oxidised cellulose gauze and sutured with absorbable sutures. If bleeding persists, locally applied tranexamic acid will be helpful. In the very unusual situation where an anticoagulated patient continues to bleed after local measures have been applied, help from a haematologist should be requested. Warfarin can be reversed with intravenous vitamin K or with fresh frozen plasma. Reversal with vitamin K is slower and has the disadvantage that there may be later resistance to warfarin. Reversal with fresh frozen plasma is immediate and does not have this problem.

Occasionally, a patient on warfarin may present as an emergency with facial injuries. In this case, the haematologist should be involved as the patient will probably need the anticoagulation reversing if there is persistent bleeding. If the patient does not appear to be actively bleeding or it has stopped, it would be prudent to inform the haematologist of the patient's existence in case a problem develops.

Sometimes an anticoagulated patient will need more extensive surgery. This is most likely to be an elderly patient who needs cancer ablation, which may involve a neck dissection where post-operative haemorrhage is potentially dangerous. Here the warfarin should be reduced over 4 or 5 days before until the INR is about 1.5. Here, the increased risk of thromboembolism will have to be accepted. In patients where the risk is highest, such as those with a recent thromboembolic event, the anticoagulation can be replaced by 'bridging therapy' with sub-cutaneous injections of low molecular weight heparin (enoxaparin). Low-molecular-weight heparin has a half-life of only a few hours and its effect can be reversed with protamine. In a very few cases, it will be necessary for the patient to receive intra-venous heparin with the dose being adjusted monitored by APPT testing.

It has been suggested that patients taking anticoagulants should not receive inferior dental nerve blocks because of the risk of serious bleeding into the medial pterygoid muscle. There has been no scientific proof that this is the case and we have never seen a case where this has been a problem.

DOAC anticoagulants and surgery

More recent direct oral anticoagulant drugs (DOAC) have been introduced which have certain advantages over warfarin for long-term anticoagulation. Dabigatran etixilate is a direct thrombin inhibitor and rivaroxaban, apixaban and edoxaban are factor 10a inhibitors. These drugs have much shorter half-lives than warfarin, so they have a more rapid onset of action after oral ingestion and a much quicker offset, provided the patient does not have renal failure. They have a lower risk of unwanted bleeding, few drug interactions, much reduced variability of effect between individuals. They do not require anticoagulant monitoring; indeed, there is no reliable test to do so. On the negative side, there is no effective way of reversing their effect other than by stopping the medication. However, idarucizumab, a newer drug which is a humanised antibody fragment, has been recently developed which binds to dabigatran and neutralises its anticoagulant effect. It can therefore be used in an emergency.

In 2012, that dabigatran received approval from the National Institute of Clinical Excellence for thrombo-prophylaxis for stroke and patients with atrial fibrillation (not accompanied by valve disease). It is therefore too soon for a definitive experience to have been established on how patients taking these drugs should be managed during surgery. However, it would appear that patients requiring dental extraction and minor oral surgery do not suffer any major problems if these drugs are continued as normal. It is recommended that ideally the surgery should be carried out 12 hours after the last dose. Wounds should be sutured and the patient should rinse with 5% tranexamic acid for a few days after the surgery.

At present, drugs for the reversal of these anticoagulants are only in development, apart from dabigatran. It would therefore be prudent that patients who need more major surgery should have them temporarily discontinued and re-started afterwards. Obviously this management should be supervised in hospital by a haematologist.

Although not anticoagulants, we would like to mention antiplatelet medication with aspirin, clopidogrel and dipyridamole. These drugs are used to prevent platelet adhesion and prevent unwanted vascular events such as acute coronary thrombosis, stroke and transient ischemic attacks. For minor oral surgery such as surgical dental extraction, the risk of bleeding which cannot be controlled by local measures is very low, so surgery should proceed without stopping the medication.

However, for more major surgery, each case should be considered on its own merit; there is little in the way of clinical trials to help firm guidelines to be formulated. If medication is to be ceased, it will need to be done several days in advance as the drugs have half-lives of several days. The decision should be made by the senior surgeon in discussion with the haematologist as sometimes this may be potentially dangerous. Some patients who have had 'drug eluting stents' fitted to prevent coronary artery occlusion are at serious risk of thrombosis if their combined aspirin and clopidogrel therapy is stopped. In such cases, the cardiologist should be involved in the decision with the consultant surgeon. You should never make the decision to stop medication yourself.

> ## _Key Points_
>
> ● For MOS for patients on Warfarin check INR is stable
>
> ● Proceed if below 4, pack wound with oxidised cellulose gauze and suture
>
> ● Patients on 'DOAC anticoagulants' proceed as normal and pack and suture as above
>
> ● Patients on clopidogrel, aspirin or dipyridamole proceed as normal for MOS
>
> ● For more major surgery involve haematologist.
>
> ● Never stop medication on your own volition

29. <u>Diabetes and Surgery</u>

With about 2.5 million diagnosed diabetics in the UK (10% type 1 & 90% type 2) plus, possibly, another half a million undiagnosed. Inevitably, you will come across some who require OMFS surgery.

Pathogenesis

You already know that diabetes mellitus is a chronic disease of carbohydrate, fat and protein metabolism. Type 1 diabetes is caused by the inability to produce insulin due to the autoimmune destruction of beta cells in the pancreas. Insulin is needed to facilitate the movement of glucose into cells from the bloodstream. Type 1 diabetes usually presents in childhood; this can be quite sudden with a ketoacidosis attack. Type 1 diabetics require lifelong insulin replacement. Type 2 usually occurs in those over 40 years, but not necessarily. Most are obese and it can initially be asymptomatic. It results from resistance to insulin, decreased insulin secretion, or excessive glucagon. Type 2 diabetics often do not need insulin replacement initially, but many will eventually.

Control

The best person to manage control of diabetes is the patient themselves, supervised by their general medical practitioner and his specialist diabetic nurse. In hospital, as much control as possible should be vested in the patient themselves within local hospital protocol. For the patient who is hitherto undiagnosed or who has poor control or complications, the specialist

---

> ### *Features of Diabetes*
>
> #### *Type 1*
>
> - Typically presents in children & young adults
> - Caused by auto-immune reaction to ß cells of islets of Langerhans cells in pancreas
> - Insulin not formed
> - Insulin needed to facilitate glucose entry to cells for energy metabolism
> - Untreated cells metabolize fat leading to release of ketones causing keto-acidosis and death
>
> #### *Type 2*
>
> - Usually presents age over 40 but not necessarily
> - Insulin level may be normal or raised but is less effective
> - Glucose level is increased but less than in type 1

> ### *Diabetic Treatment*
>
> #### *Type 1*
>
> - Typically by managing diet and exercise in conjunction with multiple injections of synthetic insulin monitored by blood glucose estimations.
> - Often twice daily insulin with longer acting synthetic insulin. Sometimes short acting insulin before food.
> - Some use subcutaneous insulin pump
>
> #### *Type 2*
>
> - Diet, exercise, weight control
> - Metformin & Thiazolidinediones (glitazones) increase the effectiveness of insulin
> - Sulphonylureas increase insulin production by pancreas
> - Eventually will need insulin

diabetic team should take control; this will include a consultant physician and a specialist nurse who will visit all in-patient diabetics daily. The anaesthetist will control the patient during the operative period. It is not the place of the surgeon to manage diabetes unguided by protocol or a specialist; and certainly not the job of the dentally qualified trainee to change or initiate treatment. So this chapter is about understanding the process of good management.

Symptoms

Most type 1 diabetics originally present with one of the following symptoms: polyuria, polydipsia, weight loss, refractory visual problems (related to osmotic changes), muscle cramps and infections. Most type 2 diabetics present with polyuria, polydipsia, candidiasis and diabetic complications (see table). However, a patient with a large dental abscess may be one of the half a million previously undiagnosed diabetics who are immunocompromised by their condition. Patients with large abscesses should therefore have their glucose levels checked.

Surgery will affect diabetic glucose control by virtue of the patient being starved for anaesthesia or by being unable to eat normally because of the surgery. Furthermore, the trauma and stress of the surgery itself will cause a stress response, leading to catabolism and hyperglycaemia and potentially

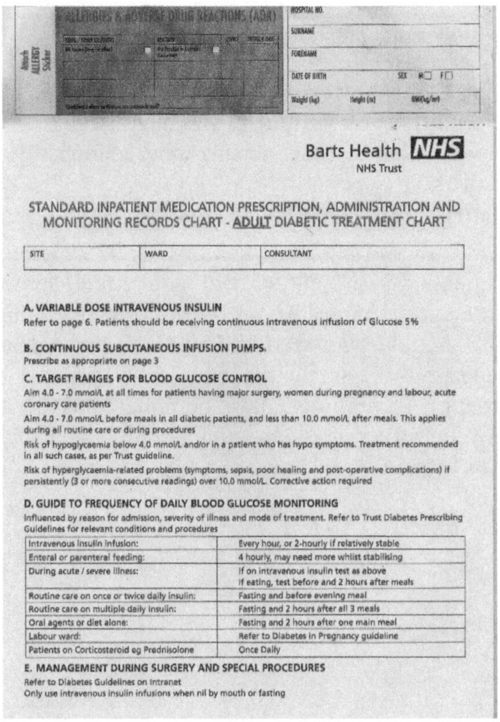

ALLERGIES & ADVERSE DRUG REACTIONS (ADR)

HOSPITAL NO.	
SURNAME	
FORENAME	
DATE OF BIRTH	SEX M☐ F☐
Weight (kg) Height (m) BMI(kg/m²)	

Barts Health NHS
NHS Trust

STANDARD INPATIENT MEDICATION PRESCRIPTION, ADMINISTRATION AND MONITORING RECORDS CHART - ADULT DIABETIC TREATMENT CHART

SITE	WARD	CONSULTANT

A. VARIABLE DOSE INTRAVENOUS INSULIN
Refer to page 6. Patients should be receiving continuous intravenous infusion of Glucose 5%

B. CONTINUOUS SUBCUTANEOUS INFUSION PUMPS.
Prescribe as appropriate on page 3

C. TARGET RANGES FOR BLOOD GLUCOSE CONTROL
Aim 4.0 - 7.0 mmol/L at all times for patients having major surgery, women during pregnancy and labour, acute coronary care patients

Aim 4.0 - 7.0 mmol/L before meals in all diabetic patients, and less than 10.0 mmol/L after meals. This applies during all routine care or during procedures

Risk of hypoglycaemia below 4.0 mmol/L and/or in a patient who has hypo symptoms. Treatment recommended in all such cases, as per Trust guideline.

Risk of hyperglycaemia-related problems (symptoms, sepsis, poor healing and post-operative complications) if persistently (3 or more consecutive readings) over 10.0 mmol/L. Corrective action required

D. GUIDE TO FREQUENCY OF DAILY BLOOD GLUCOSE MONITORING
Influenced by reason for admission, severity of illness and mode of treatment. Refer to Trust Diabetes Prescribing Guidelines for relevant conditions and procedures

Intravenous insulin infusion:	Every hour, or 2-hourly if relatively stable
Enteral or parenteral feeding:	4 hourly, may need more whilst stabilising
During acute / severe illness:	If on intravenous insulin test as above If eating, test before and 2 hours after meals
Routine care on once or twice daily insulin:	Fasting and before evening meal
Routine care on multiple daily insulin:	Fasting and 2 hours after all 3 meals
Oral agents or diet alone:	Fasting and 2 hours after one main meal
Labour ward:	Refer to Diabetes in Pregnancy guideline
Patients on Corticosteroid eg Prednisolone	Once Daily

E. MANAGEMENT DURING SURGERY AND SPECIAL PROCEDURES
Refer to Diabetes Guidelines on Intranet
Only use intravenous insulin infusions when nil by mouth or fasting

The Diabetic Treatment Chart is used to record the results of glucose estimations and prescribe subcutaneous insulin for diabetics in hospital. This is an adult chart; children will be on a paediatric ward and their diabetes will be managed by paediatricians.

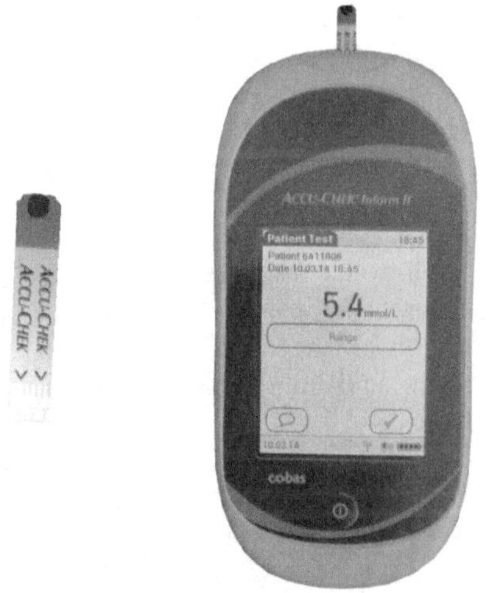

Blood glucose can be quickly tested with a blood sample taken from the end of a finger with a lancet and soaked onto a test strip (left). The strip is placed into the hand held machine (right) which gives a digital display of the result, in this case normal.

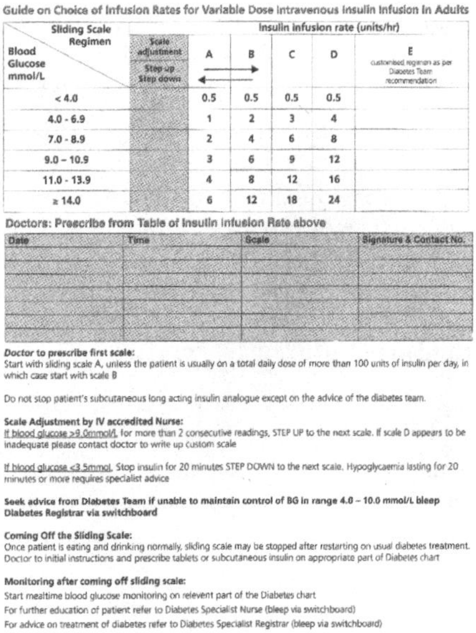

Guide on Choice of Infusion Rates for Variable Dose Intravenous Insulin Infusion in Adults

Blood Glucose mmol/L \ Sliding Scale Regimen	Scale adjustment: Step up / Step down	A	B	C	D	E customised regimen as per Diabetes Team recommendation
< 4.0		0.5	0.5	0.5	0.5	
4.0 - 6.9		1	2	3	4	
7.0 - 8.9		2	4	6	8	
9.0 – 10.9		3	6	9	12	
11.0 - 13.9		4	8	12	16	
≥ 14.0		6	12	18	24	

(Insulin infusion rate (units/hr))

Doctors: Prescribe from Table of Insulin Infusion Rate above

Date	Time	Scale	Signature & Contact No.

***Doctor* to prescribe first scale:**
Start with sliding scale A, unless the patient is usually on a total daily dose of more than 100 units of insulin per day, in which case start with scale B

Do not stop patient's subcutaneous long acting insulin analogue except on the advice of the diabetes team.

Scale Adjustment by IV accredited Nurse:
If blood glucose >9.0mmol/L for more than 2 consecutive readings, STEP UP to the next scale. If scale D appears to be inadequate please contact doctor to write up custom scale

If blood glucose <3.5mmol, Stop insulin for 20 minutes STEP DOWN to the next scale. Hypoglycaemia lasting for 20 minutes or more requires specialist advice

Seek advice from Diabetes Team if unable to maintain control of BG in range 4.0 – 10.0 mmol/L bleep Diabetes Registrar via switchboard

Coming Off the Sliding Scale:
Once patient is eating and drinking normally, sliding scale may be stopped after restarting on usual diabetes treatment. Doctor to initial instructions and prescribe tablets or subcutaneous insulin on appropriate part of Diabetes chart

Monitoring after coming off sliding scale:
Start mealtime blood glucose monitoring on relevent part of the Diabetes chart
For further education of patient refer to Diabetes Specialist Nurse (bleep via switchboard)
For advice on treatment of diabetes refer to Diabetes Specialist Registrar (bleep via switchboard)

The inside of the chart contains simple information on dosage. In practice this will probably be written up by the anaesthetist. If you are asked to prescribe you should always ask one of your medically qualified colleagues to check it.

ketoacidosis. Sepsis and inflammation reduce the effectiveness of insulin produced, making control more difficult. A type 1 insulin-dependent diabetic will typically need increased amounts of insulin in the peri-operative period or if systemically unwell. A type 2 non-insulin-dependent diabetic may need insulin to keep their glucose levels within the ideal range (6-10 mmols./litre).

Diabetes may affect the surgery, particularly in those not well controlled. Catabolism will cause delayed wound healing. There will be an increased risk of cardio-vascular complications (myocardial infarction, heart failure and stroke), and where these complications occur, mortality will be greater. Due to neuropathy, myocardial infarction is more likely to be painless. Hyperglycaemia will affect chemotaxis and phagocytosis and the function of polymorphonuclear leukocytes as well as acting as a culture medium; thus, post-operative sepsis is more likely. Although it is less likely in OMFS, diabetic patients who are immobile in bed are more likely to develop pressure sores due to small vessel disease.

Pre-op investigations

Diabetic patients presenting for cold (non-urgent) OMFS should have the standard pre-operative assessment. This will include details of any diabetic complications, how well controlled they are, and blood tests for glucose, electrolytes, and HbA1$_C$ (glycosylated haemoglobin). HbA1$_C$ is haemoglobin, which has glucose attached to it as a result of a high blood glucose. The proportion of haemoglobin, which is glycosylated, gives an indication of the blood glucose over the preceding three months (the life of a red blood cell). A level of above 69 mmols./mol. or 8.5% of total haemoglobin is considered indicative of inadequate glucose control.

Management during surgery

Many diabetics are well controlled, have no diabetic complications, and confidently monitor and manage their own glucose. If they are having a short or minor procedure and will miss only one meal, they may be admitted as a day case or have treatment under sedation. There will be a local protocol which will involve their being treated early and reducing their daily insulin (if they are to have general anaesthesia). They will need an insulin infusion with Na and KCl during surgery. In nearly every other case, they will need VRIII (variable rate intra-venous insulin infusion); this was formerly called a 'sliding scale'. There will be a separate infusion of KCl in saline and insulin with the dose varied according to hourly blood glucose levels. There will be a special chart to prescribe this and a protocol for the dose of rapidly acting insulin. The diabetic team should be informed and their specialist nurse will visit the patient daily and decide how and when they are fit to be weaned back onto their normal regime.

Hypoglycemia

●Caused by too much insulin, inadequate food intake, exercise, stress, alcohol
●Can occur quickly
●Most diabetics can recognise symptoms: sweating, shakiness, tachycardia, anxiety
●Brain most susceptible as unable to metabolize fat leading to unconsciousness
●Quickly responds to oral glucose or, if unconscious, glucagon injection
●Well controlled diabetics are less able to recognize symptoms

Hyperglycemia

●Associated with low intracellular glucose
●Cells metabolize fat for energy producing ketones
●Ketones are toxic and cause acidosis
●Diabetic ketoacidosis is dangerous and causes death

Complications of Diabetes

●**Large vessel arteriosclerosis**: myocardial infarction, stroke, peripheral vascular disease
●**Small vessel disease***: nephropathy, retinopathy, cataracts.
●**Neuropathy:** peripheral, autonomic

Patients who present for cold (non-urgent) surgery who are poorly controlled or have high glucose or high HbA1$_C$ should be referred to their GP for advice and management. Diabetic patients who present as emergency admissions, have complications or are poorly controlled should be monitored by the diabetic team as routine.

Key Points

● Contact diabetic team for undiagnosed diabetes or those with poor control or complications

●For cold (non-urgent) OMFS surgery – standard preoperative assessment and check HbA1c for recent glucose control

●For well controlled diabetes – consult local protocol – inform diabetic team - variable rate intravenous insulin infusion (VRIII) or 'sliding scale', KCl in saline and hourly blood glucose check – special chart

●For poorly controlled diabetes – refer to their GP for management or diabetic physician

---

30. Medication Related Osteonecrosis of the Jaws (MRONJ)

We first started seeing cases of MRONJ in 2002 which were related to the use of bisphosphonate medication to treat malignant bone metastases. This appeared to be a new disease but in fact was exactly the same as that of the 19th century caused by phosphorus used in the manufacture of matches and particularly described in the match workers of London's East End and, described by Dickens. Then it was called 'phossy jaw'.

Although initially it appeared to be caused solely by bisphosphonates − which inhibit osteoclastic function − and so was called bisphosphonate related osteonecrosis, it was later found that other anti-resorptive or anti-angiogenic drugs can cause it; hence, the present name.

The disease is defined as necrotic bone exposed in the maxillofacial region for more than 8 weeks in patients previously treated with bisphosphonates or anti-resorptive agents who have not received radiotherapy.

Use of bisphosphonates

Most cases we see are caused by bisphosphonates. They are prescribed in low doses in oral form for patients with osteopenia and osteoporosis, mostly post-menopausal women, to prevent pathological fractures. It is used in higher dose through intermittent intra-venous infusions for the management of Paget's disease of bone, hypercalcaemia of malignancy, multiple myeloma and for skeletal metastases. It is used most commonly in women with breast cancer and also men with prostate cancer. Osteopenia and osteoporosis are common in post-menopausal women and particularly predispose to fractured neck of femur, an event which can be fatal in the frail. Many elderly ladies will be prescribed bisphosphonates when they have steroids for whatever reason, as steroids decrease bone density.

Bisphosphonate action

The drugs work mainly by inhibiting osteoclastic bone resorption. They accumulate in bone, particularly where there is a high bone turnover, as in the alveolus of the jaws. They may also inhibit tumour cells invading bone and cause tumour cell death. It is possible that bisphosphonate may be released from bone by the trauma of dental extractions and thus inhibit soft tissue healing; they may also decrease intra-bony blood circulation. There is a very high turnover of bone during

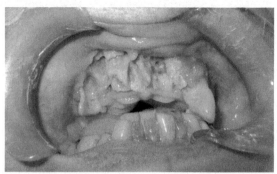

This lady presented with exposed bone in her maxilla a few weeks after she had 3 incisors removed. She has taken oral bisphosphonates along with prednisolone for polymyalgia. When she had the teeth removed it had been some time since she had taken the medication and had forgotten about it. Over the following 9 months her whole maxilla sloughed out.

remodelling after dental extraction, so that symptoms are most likely to develop in this circumstance.

Denosumab, not a bisphosphonate, interferes with osteoclast function and has been used for post-menopausal osteoporosis and, in some cases, replacing bisphosphonate for cancer patients. Bevacizumab and sunitinib may be used in combination with bisphosphonates; they also contribute to necrosis.

Incidence and prevalence

The best estimate of the incidence of the problem is of perhaps 10 patients in a million per year. Patients taking the medication orally for osteoporosis or osteopenia (most commonly alendronic acid) are considered to be at low risk but the risk increases with the length of time they are taking the medication. The time of onset of the disease is usually over 4 years from starting to take the medication for these patients and after 5 years, the low risk patients are considered to now be at high risk. Anyone taking steroids is as well is considered to be at high risk.

Those taking higher dose bisphosphonates by intermittent infusions (most commonly zoledronic acid) are considered higher risk. They would normally get problems after more than 3 years of therapy. However, there are more patients with problems related to oral ingestion than IV infusion because of the much larger number prescribed the former.

Although the incidence is rare, you will see a significant number of these patients in OMFS

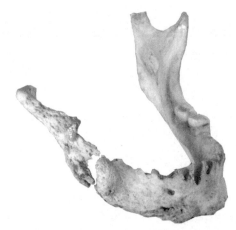

19th century mandible from match worker with phosphorus jaw necrosis. Courtesy of Royal College of Surgeons of England.

Charles Dickens wrote these words in his journal 'Household Words' in 1852. He was describing 'phossy jaw' which affected workers exposed to phosphorus in the match industry. It was exactly the same disease as phosphorus necrosis caused by bisphosphonates 150 years later.

departments as the medication is prescribed for chronic problems and patients return quite often with infective exacerbations. This applies to even the patients with metastatic breast cancer. Modern therapy and bisphosphonate means that ladies with metastatic breast cancer can lead normal lives for years. Whatever the complications (which only a small proportion get) they are wonderful drugs; hitherto metastatic breast cancer would have been crippling.

Symptoms

Bone necrosis itself can be asymptomatic but when it becomes infected, swelling, pain and discharge develop. In most cases, this is precipitated by dental extraction, although it can occur from denture trauma, particularly on the thin mucosa lingually in the lower molar area or over tori. The longer a patient has been on the medication, the greater the risk; most of those on oral bisphosphonate have taken it for three years before getting symptoms. Symptoms can progress to chronic fistulae discharging into the mouth or extra-orally. The necrotic bone can extend beyond the alveolar bone and lead to oro-antral or oro-nasal communication of pathological fracture.

Management

The Scottish Dental Clinical Effectiveness programme has produced guidelines on the dental management of patients taking these medications. Patients should be made dentally fit before starting the drugs. Your hospital may have a fast track system for patients to be assessed before they start medication (particularly IV) and any non-restorable teeth removed and the socket allowed to heal for three weeks before the first dose. Our experience has shown that OMFS referral and subsequent treatment prior to bisphosphonate therapy keeps the risk of bone necrosis low.

Good oral hygiene support and restorative care should be provided by someone, and smoking should be advised against. Patients on oral bisphosphonates are at lower risk, especially if taking the drug for a short time. They may have extractions carried out as atraumatically as possible and sharp socket edges burred back without raising a muco-periosteal flap. These low-risk patients can have any simple extractions carried out in primary care, but dental practitioners may be reluctant to carry out more complicated surgical extractions and these may be referred into a hospital.

Patients taking oral drugs for over three years, and particularly those taking steroids, should be warned of higher risk. It has been considered that cessation of the bisphosphonates may be helpful, but the drugs bind to bone so well that it is considered that stopping for anything less than a year before extractions would probably not be helpful. Denosumab does not bind into the skeleton like bisphosphonates, so ceasing the drug will allow the effect on osteoclasts to recover so that its effects are reversible in time. Stopping steroids is considered to produce an immediate reduction in risk and if this is not possible, then reducing the dose to below 7.5 mg. per day may help. Preoperative chlorhexidine mouth rinses or antibiotics are not recommended unless there is active sepsis present. Patients on IV bisphosphonates should avoid

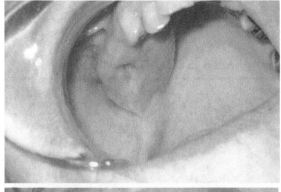

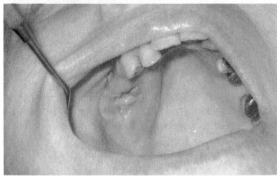

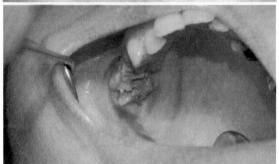

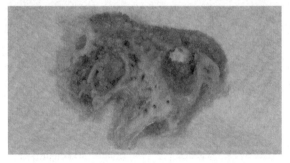

A typical case. This lady was able to have a normal lifestyle for many years in spite of metastatic breast cancer thanks to her monthly bisphosphonate infusions. She presented with discharge after removal of her upper first molar. The images show the alveolar bone extruding over a period of 2 years. After the socket was exfoliated pus continued to discharge.

extractions wherever feasible. For unrestorable teeth, removing the crown and root filling the root has been advocated.

Patients who have osteonecrosis may be asymptomatic with exposed bone in the mouth. Some have advocated covering exposed bone with local flaps but they should be managed as conservatively as possible, keeping the area clean with chlorhexidine without brushing the delicate soft tissues and exposing more bone. When the exposed bone becomes infected, they will get swelling, pain, discharge and halitosis. Acute exacerbations may be managed with penicillin based antibiotics, or metronidazole. Bone concentrating antibiotics such as tetracycline or clindamycin may be useful. However, chronic sepsis for months or years is the norm; if the sepsis is draining it may be painless, just sore. Some may advocate removing large bony sequestra and infected necrotic bone and covering with local flaps, but surgery may increase the risk of pathological fracture.

In cases where the mandible is discharging pus extra-orally or where there is a pathological fracture, a segmental resection of the mandible and reconstruction with vascularised free flaps may be considered.

Reference See:

Scottish Dental Clinical Effectiveness Programme: Oral Health Management of Patients at Risk of Medication-related Osteonecrosis of the Jaw (2017). Search online and download.

31. Introduction to Orthognathic Surgery

Correction of facial deformity can be complicated and involve various surgical procedures. Craniofacial surgery, which involves high level facial osteotomies on syndromic youngsters, is normally carried out in a few craniofacial units which have sufficient case numbers to maintain the specialist expertise. However, orthognathic surgery (correction of jaw disproportion) is common, fairly simple and carried out in most OMFS departments with one operation, the bimaxillary osteotomy. This comprises a maxillary osteotomy at Le Fort 1 level and a sagittal split osteotomy of the mandible (Bimax).

Indications for surgery

There are a handful of cases carried out to improve the airway in patients with obstructive sleep apnoea. However, most cases will be young adults who have a severe bony discrepancy in their dental base relationships and a malocclusion which cannot be corrected by orthodontics alone.

The whole process will involve many orthodontic visits besides a major surgical operation. A lot of commitment is needed both from the patient and their family. The patients are highly motivated, as they are expecting an improvement in facial appearance besides a functional occlusion with stable oral health. Many youngsters with facial or jaw disproportion will be affected psychologically by their appearance and may have experienced teasing or bullying at school. Some OMFS departments may have a clinical psychologist attached to their teams, but we are unsure of what the benefit.

Patterns of jaw discrepancy

Most cases will follow one of two patterns: the class 3 cases, which are the most common, and the class 2 division 1. In the class 3 cases, the mandible will be prognathic compared to the maxilla. The maxillary buccal segments will be too narrow, and the upper incisors will be proclined towards the mandibular incisors which will be retroclined by the soft tissues towards the maxillary. The incisor relationship will be class 3 or just edge to edge. Facially, the patient will have an obviously prominent mandible. The maxilla will appear flat in profile and long so that there will be more than the ideal 2 mm incisor show when the mouth is at rest. The patient may show too much gingiva when smiling rather than the lip moving only to the gingival margin.

Class 3 case before orthodontics

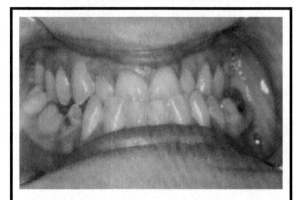

Pre-treatment. There is a reverse overjet with the lower incisors in front of the uppers and the lower buccal segments are wider than the upper.

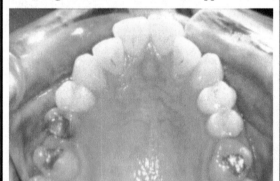

Pre-treatment. The upper arch is irregular.

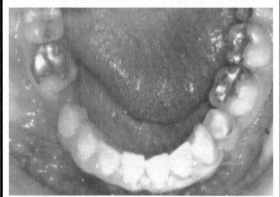

Pre-treatment. The lower incisors are obviously retroclined as well as there being irregularities.

In the class 2 division 1 cases the patient will have an obvious mandibular deficiency in profile with upper incisors proclined by the lower lip which fits inside them and over-erupted lower incisors producing a significantly increased curve of Spee to the occlusion; the lower incisors may traumatise the palatal gingiva.

Pre-operative orthodontics

Children with bony jaw discrepancies should be seen by the orthodontist early, as they can often influence growth patterns using treatment with extra-oral headgear. In cases where the patient will need surgery to correct their disproportion, they should be seen by the orthodontist and surgeon together with their parents before surgery is contemplated. A dental examination, orthopantomograph and lateral

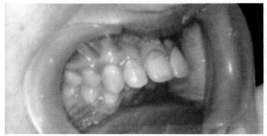

Class 2 div. 1

cephalometric X-rays are carried out and study models taken. After these examinations, the recommendations concerning possible surgery can be made and considered by the patient. These steps are normally carried out over several visits. When recommendations are made, it is essential that the patient is informed of all the potential complications and side effects of the treatment, both orthodontic and surgical. Consent for the treatment is obtained and recorded in writing. It is helpful if all this information is put in writing, as a letter to the patient, with copies to the primary care practitioners, and a copy kept with the written confirmation of consent. We like to introduce the patient to meet someone who has already undergone surgery.

Apart from an orthopantomograph X-ray, a lateral cephalometric X-ray is made. This involves an image taken with the X-ray source some distance away from the patient and sensor so that the rays are near parallel. This image can then be traced to measure angles of the face and dentition and facial height, and to predict the result for the patient. However, we have some reservations about prediction as it is not always accurate. We are nervous about disappointing a patient if the appearance is not as they feel they had been promised. It is imperative that before orthodontics is

started that the patient is motivated to achieve high standards of oral hygiene and sensible diet as the pre-surgical orthodontics will take between one and two years with fixed appliances.

In the common class 3 cases the aim of orthodontics is to correct any irregularity in the occlusion, expand the maxillary buccal segments and de-compensate the incisor tilting. The upper incisor angulation should be near the normal 109° to the maxillary plane and the lower incisors are 90° to the mandibular plane. This will make the facial appearance worse initially; the patient should have been warned about it.

In class 2 cases, where the mandible is to be moved forward, the orthodontics will also need to help flatten the curve of Spee and tilt the incisors in the opposite direction to that of a class 3 case. If the lower incisors have erupted significantly, then the lower labial segment may be set down at surgery in which case orthodontics can create a small space between the canines and premolars to make room for a bone cut. Surgery for class 2 cases sometimes involves a genioplasty to put the chin forward to help mask the skeletal discrepancy, if this is severe.

Surgery

The surgery, which results in discomfort (rather than frank pain), difficulty eating, some time with jaws held together, and a change in appearance, is a major life event for most. It is frequently carried out at the age of 17 when growth has finished. In order that it should interfere with education as little as possible, this is often at the end of the school year, before the start of higher education. The end of June through to the beginning of August is a busy time for the orthognathic surgeon. Treatment will normally involve 12 – 24 months of pre-surgical orthodontics followed by surgery and approximately 6 months of orthodontic retention before everything is complete.

Before the orthodontics has been completed, the patient should be seen again by a surgeon and a date set for surgery. The procedure should be explained to them again and they should be warned about side effects and complications and the final movements are planned. The orthodontist will order a new lateral cephalometric X-ray image which will be traced digitally to help with the planning, and new study models will be made to be mounted on an articulator.

Planning surgery

Generally, the orthodontist will prescribe the movements to be made using the cephalometric tracings

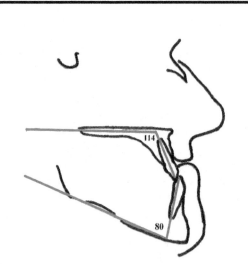

Before: The soft tissues have 'compensated' the incisor relationship for the discrepancy in the dental base relationship. The tongue has tilted the upper incisors forward to an angulation of 114° to the maxillary plane (norm: 109°) and the lip has tilted the lower incisor back to an angulation of 80° to the mandibular plane (norm: 90°).

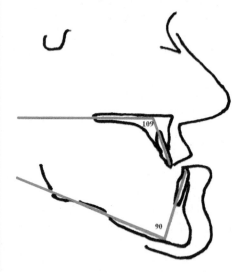

After: The incisors have been 'decompensated' to the normal angulation ready for surgery. The patient should be warned of the temporary adverse effect on facial profile.

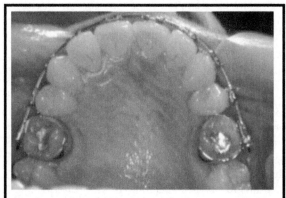

The upper arch has been expanded and irregularities removed. The incisors have been retroclined towards the norm of 108° to the maxillary plane.

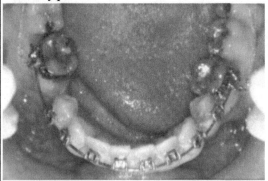

The lower incisors have been inclined forward to bring the lower incisor to mandibular place angle towards the norm of 90°.

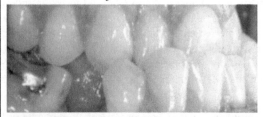

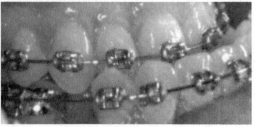

After pre-surgical orthodontics the incisor relation will look worse (above before, below after).

to analyse the facial skeleton. However, any competent OMFS surgeon will be able to prescribe the movements to be made from clinical examination as follows:-

1. First look at the patient in profile and see if there is any flat appearance of the face (para-nasal flattening) and what the angle is between the upper lip and alar of the nose (90° norm). 2. Decide if the maxilla needs to be advanced to get the optimal facial appearance: not at all, a little (3mm), a medium amount (6 mm) or a lot (9 mm). 3. Observe the face from in front: does it look long? Observe the amount of incisor show with the lips at rest (2 mm norm) and when the patient is smiling (lips to top of clinical crown). This assumes a normal lip length of 22 mm for males and 20 mm for females. Then decide if the maxilla needs to be impacted surgically, not at all, a little (2mms), a medium amount (4 mm) or a lot (6 mm).

We like to compare our conclusion made by clinical examination with that of the orthodontists made radiographically; the result is nearly always within a mm or so. It is a nonsense to measure differential distances in single millimetres; the surgical technique is simply not that accurate.

Model Surgery

The models are then mounted on an articulator by the technician, who then carries out model surgery to the maxilla and makes the prescribed movements and constructs a wafer to fit between the teeth after the maxilla has been moved and before the mandible. This ''intermediate wafer' is used by the surgeon to position the maxilla after making the cuts, while it is plated firmly into position. The mandible is then moved into a class 1 relationship to the maxilla and a wafer made to hold the mandible firmly in position with the jaws wired together while the surgeon plates the mandible.

Surgery and orthodontic retention

Surgery takes from just over an hour for a single jaw operation and up to four and a half hours for a bimaxillary procedure. Patients should be warned that they may need up to three nights in hospital, but in practice, only one is normally required.

Although the jaws are plated with titanium plates, they are normally approximated together with inter-maxillary elastic bands. This is done because the patient will have to re-learn the proprioception necessary to close the mandible into a correct occlusive position. The elastics may be placed the day

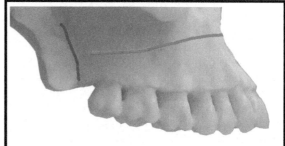

The pterygoid plates are disconnected from the maxilla with a curved chisel placed behind the maxilla (blue line), the buccal maxilla is cut with a bur or saw through the lateral wall of the nose (anteriorly) and lateral wall of antrum (posteriorly-red line) and the nasal septum is divided with a chisel using only hand pressure (not shown).

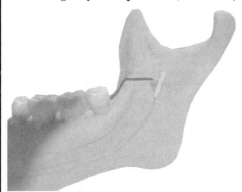

The mandible cortex is cut medially (red line) through to bleeding cancellous bone within just above the lingua, so avoiding the ID bundle (yellow), and only half way back and is continued down the external oblique ridge buccally.

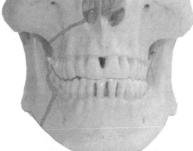

The cortical cut is extended down and through the cortical bone at the lower border. The cuts top and bottom are then gently opened with a large chisel and the maxilla downfractured and the mandible split sagittally.

after the operation or a few days later at the first followup appointment. Patients are normally given steroids during the peri-operative period. This helps reduce the amount of oedematous swelling, reduce nausea and the amount of analgesia needed. It also delays swelling, so they must be warned that they will swell further in the couple of days following surgery before it starts to go down. Once surgery is over, the patient will probably need a few further months with an orthodontic appliance to help retain the teeth in the new positions.

Relapse

One of the potential complications of this type of surgery is relapse. That is the soft tissues, muscles, ligaments have a habit of pulling the bony skeleton back to where it used to be. Patients should be warned that in many cases there will be a very small amount of relapse in the years after surgery, but in a very few cases, the relapse may be more significant. Having a well-fitting positive occlusion will help stability, as will keep the movements to a minimum by equalising the correction of the discrepancy between both maxilla and mandible. Thus, in most cases, patients will have surgery to both jaws: the 'bimax'.

We hope you will be able to participate in the treatment of orthognathic patients. You should make sure you interview and examine any patient whose operation you assist with and be able to see them in the clinic during the post-operative period.

With increasing specialisation, there are now many surgeons who do little other than orthognathic surgery; this has the advantage that they can offer less frequently performed operations for more unusual deformities. The vast majority of cases, however, continue to be managed with simple 'bimax'.

Side effects of surgery

Swelling
Bruising
Jaws fixed together
Discomfort eating
Weight Loss
Temporary numbness or tingling of lip or chin

Complications of Surgery

Permanent numbness of lip or chin (approx 30%)
Relapse
Infection of bone plates necessitating surgery for removal

Class 3 case before (left) and after (right)

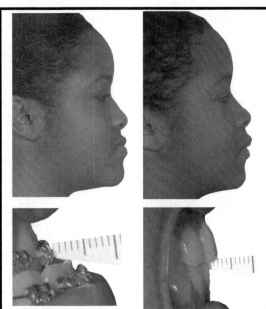

Pre-treatment the mandible is prognathic, the maxilla looks slightly flat beside the nose, there is a reverse overjet of 3 mms.

Class 2 case before (left) and after (right)

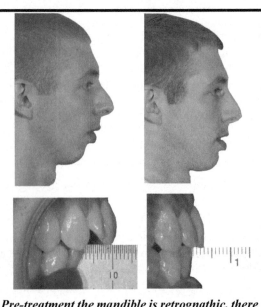

Pre-treatment the mandible is retrognathic, there is an overjet of 9 mms.

32. <u>Management of Salivary Gland Swellings</u>

You should expect to see a good number of swellings of the salivary glands in any OMFS department. These will mostly be caused by obstruction to the outflow of saliva from the glands and less commonly caused by tumours, most of which will be benign.

Mucous cysts

Most common are mucoceles in the lower lip. Mucoceles are pseudocysts (no lining) that consist of saliva which has extravasated into the surrounding soft tissues usually consequent upon damage to the salivary gland ducts by the teeth. Their treatment is removal of the gland, which feeds the swelling. The procedure requires exposing the small mucous glands via a vertical incision within the oral mucosa. There are multiple small nerves ascending to the vermillion of the lower lip which can be damaged during the procedure, leading to numbness. It is easy to miss removing the precise small gland causing the swelling. This is not a procedure to be carried out by someone inexperienced.

A ranula is a mucocele of the sublingual salivary gland. This is usually seen as a soft swelling in the floor of the mouth. Occasionally, the swelling may penetrate below the mylohyoid muscle into the neck and be seen as a soft swelling in the submandibular area. This is called a plunging ranula, but the principal of treatment is the same.

Surgery for a ranula is therefore removal of the sublingual gland, but access is difficult so that a general anaesthetic is nearly always indicated. The sublingual gland is shaped like a tadpole with the thinner end forming into the duct, which is closely associated with the deep part of the submandibular gland. It does not normally shell out easily; it is more like a controlled

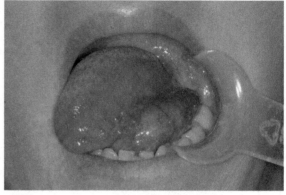

Ranula

tearing and there is a risk of damage to the lingual nerve and duct of the submandibular gland. Furthermore, there is a healthy network of vessels in the floor of the mouth, which can result in prolonged bleeding. Removal of the roof of the ranula under local anaesthetic will relieve the symptoms in the short term, but it is likely to recur. However, in children the chances of recurrence are much less and this may often be used as a definitive treatment.

Salivary obstruction

Strictures or, more commonly, stones in the ducts of the submandibular glands can cause swelling associated with eating. The resulting salivary stasis can lead to painful ascending infection - sialadentis. The submandibular gland is more frequently involved than the parotid. Removal of a stone which is causing obstruction from the duct in the floor of the mouth may be relatively straightforward under local anaesthetic if it is located anteriorly. This can produce immediate relief of symptoms, but there may be other stones in the gland, which may cause problems in the future. These may sometimes show up on plain

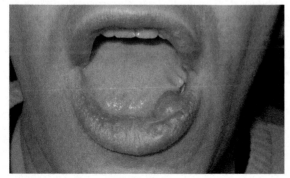

A typical mucocoele in the lip

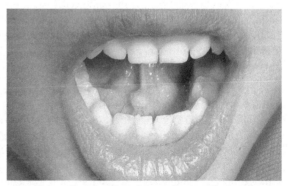

A stone at the papilla of the submandibular duct

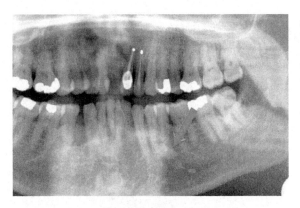

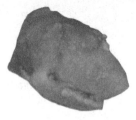

Some stones may be seen on X-ray as in this OPG above, otherwise ultrasound imaging is most reliable. Below the stone after removal.

radiographs but are better demonstrated by an ultrasound scan. After removal of a stone from the duct, the wound should be left open, and the patient encouraged to stimulate saliva to decrease the likelihood of stricture formation in the duct.

A submandibular gland, which has experienced obstruction and recurrent sialadentis over a prolonged period, will probably need its removal to prevent further symptoms. Patients who get immediate relief from removal of a stone from the floor of the mouth should be warned that such surgery may be needed at some time in the future.

Obstruction of the outflow of the parotid gland may be because of a stricture more commonly than a stone. This may be demonstrated with sialography, where a radiopaque contrast is injected into the duct to enable an image of the ductal system to be made. This may be therapeutic as well as diagnostic as it may flush out plugs of mucous which are causing obstruction.

Less frequently, a stone may be formed in the parotid gland and cause obstruction in the duct by coming to rest at the papilla. Incising the papilla over the stone may produce scarring leading to a stricture later. This risk may be minimised by making a C-shaped incision over the stone behind the papilla to remove the stone and to leave it open to drain. A stone

which is mobile rather than stuck may be removed by basket retrieval. A very thin wire is passed into the duct of the gland, a plunger is pressed and the basket opens up and is withdrawn, pulling the stone with it. This may be used concurrently with a sialo-endoscope, which enables the inside of the duct to be visualised; it has the advantage of not using radiation. Sometimes strictures of the parotid may be relieved (at least temporarily) by dilation with an arterial balloon catheter.

Salivary tumours

Salivary gland tumours are most common in the parotid gland. Pleomorphic adenoma is the commonest; although benign, it can increase in size slowly over several years and spread beyond the capsule of the gland and therefore need to be removed with a margin of normal tissue, as with a malignant tumour. If not completely removed with a margin, they have a propensity to recur several years later and seed in several different parts of the face and become very difficult to control in the long term. They can also give rise to a malignant tumour from the benign tissue. The typical operation for removal of pleomorphic adenoma is removal of all the superficial parotid gland, i.e. all the gland superficial to the facial nerve, which is about 80% of the total volume of the gland. Tumours arising in the 20% deep part of the gland are rare.

Warthin's tumours are the next most common, also benign. It is not essential to remove them, but if they are visible on the face, they may be removed for cosmesis. Warthins can be bilateral and can sometimes cause pain, which would be an indication for removal; they most frequently affect women and are associated with smoking.

Tumours of the submandibular gland and sublingual glands are much less common than of the parotid, but when they do occur are more likely to be malignant. There are several types of malignant salivary gland tumours, but the least uncommon are mucoepidermoid, adenocystic and adenocarcinoma. Mucoepidermoid carcinomas come in different grades of malignancy; some behave fairly innocuously, being more like benign tumours, with the higher grade ones behaving like a squamous cancer. Adenocystic carcinomas are malignant but tend to grow very slowly and have a propensity to grow along nerves. They have a very good 5 year survival rate but tend to recur many years later while adenocarcinomas behave as classical malignant tumours.

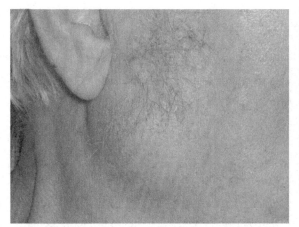

A parotid lump. Most likely a pleomorphic adenoma in the superficial part of the gland. Examination should include checking the external ear and side of head for skin cancer least this be metastatic cancer in intra-parotid lymph nodes and facial nerve function which will always be normal with benign tumour. The suspected diagnosis should be confirmed by fine needle aspiration cytology and an ultrasound scan or CT will demonstrate the extent of the tumour.

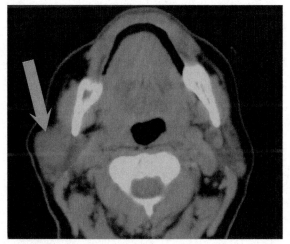

A parotid is defined in the superficial parotid by computerised tomography (CT)

Salivary gland removal

The operation you are most likely to see for salivary tumours is superficial parotidectomy. The parotid gland superficial to the facial nerve where most of the tumours originate is removed usually through an incision just anterior to the pinna of the ear. The facial nerve is identified as it leaves the stylomastoid foramen and followed forward, leaving it intact but removing the gland superficial to it. Afterwards, the patient can expect temporary facial nerve weakness because the nerve has been

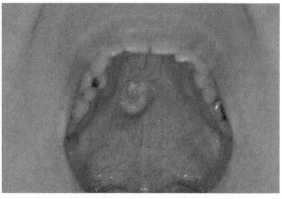

Occasionally tumours may arise in minor salivary glands. This is a pleomorphic adenoma.

manipulated, but this can be expected to recover, assuming the nerve has not been cut. Permanent facial nerve paralysis is very deforming. The affected side of the face will droop, which will be progressive, as tone is lost from the facial muscles. Many patients will exhibit Frey's syndrome (gustatory sweating) after parotidectomy. They will experience sweating on the side of the face as secretomotor fibres from the gland stimulate sweat glands in the skin. Patients should be warned before surgery.

Removal of the submandibular gland is a fairly straightforward operation approached through a skin crease below the mandible to give the best cosmesis. The incision should be low enough to avoid the mandibular branch of the facial nerve. The gland is normally shelled out quite easily unless there has been prolonged sialadentis causing fibrosis; the duct of the gland is tied before being cut. The lingual nerve which crosses the duct should be observed and preserved. Access to the sublingual gland is from the floor of the mouth but its removal is awkward as it does not shell out easily and the submandibular gland duct and lingual nerve can potentially be damaged.

Imaging

Imaging for swellings is primarily by ultrasound. This will tell the clinician whether the swelling is multifocal, bilateral, the size and whether it originates in the salivary tissue or in the lymph glands within the parotid gland, which may be enlarged by metastatic squamous cancer from the skin.

33. <u>Benign Odontogenic Cysts and Tumours</u>

Odontogenic cysts are either inflammatory secondary to dental disease or developmental. We have listed these.

We do not think it necessary for you to be familiar with the behaviour of the rare odontogenic tumours for your clinical work, or for non-specialist dental examinations. However, it is necessary to know that the commonest two, ameloblastoma and keratocyst, may present in the same way as an odontogenic cyst. These are benign and do not metastasise, but they do invade locally. The keratocyst has been reclassified as 'keratocystic odontogenic tumour', but it is still widely referred to as a cyst. It is cystic but behaves aggressively.

Odontogenic cysts

Most cysts present as a radiolucency on an x-ray image with a distinct dense periphery where the bone has reacted to the pressure of the expanding cyst. The most common will be a radicular cyst caused by dentally induced inflammation in a granuloma at the apex of a non-vital tooth. These will enlarge slowly over several years and eventually can reach a size large enough to penetrate the cortical bone. They may then become infected, which is when the patient will present

---

Odontogenic Inflammatory Cysts

Radicular: Most common; at apex of dead tooth; formed from epithelial rests in granuloma stimulated by inflammation from tooth

Residual: Radicular cyst after tooth removed

Paradental: Rare; are lateral to tooth from periodontal inflammation of the epithelial rests

Odontogenic Developmental Cysts

Dentigerous Cyst: Next common to radicular; surrounds crown of unerupted tooth; most usually upper canine or lower third molar; forms from the dental follicle

Eruption Cyst: Dentigerous cyst over crown of erupting tooth; ruptures as tooth erupts

Lateral Periodontal Cyst: Lateral or between roots of a vital tooth; arises from odontogenic epithelial remnants

Gingival Cyst: Arises from dental lamina rests; similar to lateral periodontal cyst; more common in infants where it resolves spontaneously; rare in adults where it needs removal

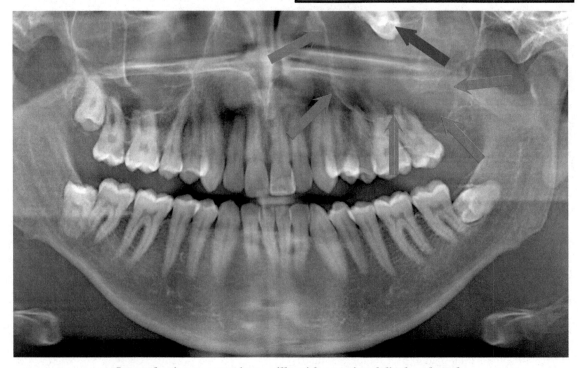

Large dentigerous cyst in maxilla with associated displaced tooth

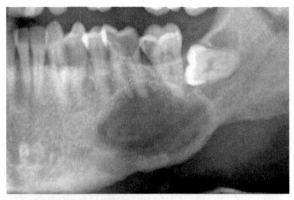

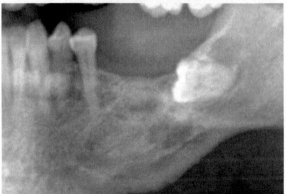

Above: radicular cyst related to dead lower first molar, found on x-ray, no symptoms.
Below: one year post operation the cyst cavity has filled with woven bone and is slowly maturing towards normality

for treatment if they have not already been found from a routine dental x-ray. X-rays will show the lesion to be unilocular and there will be no resorption of the teeth.

The second most common cyst is the developmental dentigerous cyst. This occurs most commonly in the third molar region of the mandible. It will be seen on x-ray as a radiolucent lesion enveloping the crown of an erupted tooth.

Surgical management of cysts

It is normal for a provisional diagnosis to be made based on the clinical and x-ray appearance. Standard treatment is surgical enucleation; the cyst is shelled out, preferably without fragmenting it, to improve the change of leaving no part of the cyst lining behind. We usually aspirate the cyst at the beginning of the operation to deflate it and facilitate its removal from the bone. Aspiration helps with diagnosis. A keratocyst will have a very thick fluid containing keratin, whereas other cysts have a much thinner fluid within. Very

Benign Epithelial Odontogenic Tumours
Commoner:

Ameloblastoma: Locally aggressive; need surgical clearance of one cm; do not metastasise; large irregular bone cavity; expands cortical bone but it unusually penetrates through it; usually multiloculated

Keratocystic Odontogenic Tumour [Keratocyst] Most commonly known as keratocyst; very thin lining; thick cyst fluid containing keratin; usually multiloculated; wall has 'daughter cysts' and epithelial proliferation; high recurrence rate if parakeratinised lining; lower recurrence if orthokeratinised lining (rarer); tends not to expand cortex so spreads widely before presenting late; bony cavity should be curetted 1-2 mms to reduce recurrence

Rarer:

Calcifying Epitheloid Odontogenic (Pindborg) Tumour: penetrates cancellous bone and expands cortex; does not penetrate cortex; may contain a tooth; behaves like ameloblastoma but can be mistaken for a malignancy; local excision with a margin of bone is adequate

Adenomatoid Odontogenic Tumour: Presents as a cyst which envelops the crown of a tooth

Squamous Odontogenic tumour: Consists of squamous epithelium which degenerates into cystic cavities; calcification may occur; can infiltrate cancellous bone and loosen teeth

Benign Mixed Epithelial & Connective Tissue Odontogenic Tumour

Ameloblastic fibroma: usually occurs in teens; slow growing & destructive; presents as a cyst; expands jaw; cured by complete removal

Benign Connective Tissue Odontogenic Tumours

Odontogenic fibroma; a slow growing fibrous mass; usually in mandible; removal is usually easy and is curative

Odontogenic myxoma: occurs in the young; loose mucoid material infiltrates widely; should be removed with a wide margin; may recur years later

Cementoblastoma: usually seen in young; benign radiopacity at apex of mandibular molar surrounded by a lucency; should be removed with the tooth occasionally, a vascular lesion will present as a cyst and the procedure should be abandoned, and the patient sent for embolisation before proceeding. The wound should be closed primarily and the margins of the flap must be positioned well away from the cyst over sound bone. This reduces the risk of the wound breaking down.

Smaller lesions, particularly in the anterior maxilla, can be removed with local anaesthesia. Larger lesions, in areas where surgical access is more difficult, are more usually done with general anaesthesia.

The mucosa over large cyst cavities has a tendency to breakdown during healing. This risk can be reduced by ensuring that the wound margin is cut well away from the cyst cavity on healthy bone. Very large cyst cavities which are more liable to break down may be packed with a disinfectant dressing of Whitehead's varnish or BIPP on ribbon gauze. This will protect the cavity from ingress of food. The pack is then shortened in stages so that the cavity gradually heals from its base. Healing will be prolonged, but should be cleaner and more comfortable.

Aggressive cysts and odontogenic tumours

There are certain features of a cystic lesion which suggest a keratocyst, ameloblastoma or one of the rarer odontogenic tumours. These need more radical treatment than a radicular or dentigerous cyst. These features are: rapid expansion of the cortical bone, large size, multi-locular appearance on the x-ray and loosening or resorption of the adjacent teeth.

In these circumstances, we usually carry out a biopsy for histopathology. With a keratocyst, we will find a very thin cavity lining and a very thick keratin containing fluid, which makes the diagnosis immediately obvious. The pathologist should always have the facility to look at the x-ray image to help in diagnosis.

For a keratocyst, ameloblastoma or several of the rarer odontogenic tumours, a more aggressive operation will be needed than for a radicular or dentigerous cyst. Keratocysts may have small 'daughter cysts' arising from their linings; because of this and a higher mitotic activity in their linings, they tend to recur. They must therefore be removed with a 1-2 mm margin of bone from around them. A technique we like is after removal of all the soft tissue to paint the bony margin of the cyst cavity with methylene blue. This penetrates the bone to a depth of 2 mm. The blue dye is then removed with a rotating bur so that the operator can be confident that the cavity has been

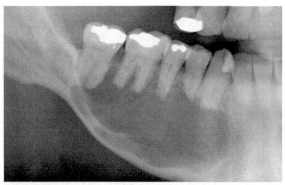

Detail from an OPG shows a suspicious multifollicular cystic cavity of mandible with tooth resorption. This appearance would induce us to carry out a biopsy before planning surgery. It was an ameloblastoma

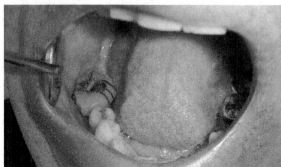

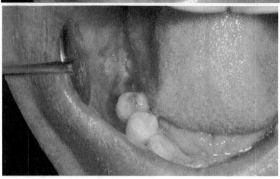

Top: the above ameloblastoma has been biopsied and a decompression stent placed to marsupialise the lesion. Below: a few weeks later the stent is removed, the lesion is smaller and can be managed with less destructive surgery

curetted to a satisfactory depth for clearance of all residual cells.

An ameloblastoma and some of the other odontogenic tumours will need a much more radical approach, but not as radical as for an invasive cancer. Bone should be removed with a one centimetre clearance around the tumour. This might involve a marginal resection of the mandible with bone graft reconstruction. In some cases, complete resection of a portion of the mandible and reconstruction with a free vascularized bone graft will be needed, as we do for a cancer, but without such as large resection margin.

Marsupialisation is a technique we can use for very large cysts or for smaller lesions to avoid a more substantial operation, as it might be done with local anaesthetic if in an accessible area of the mouth. A window of bone and the cyst lining are removed, but the rest of the lesion is left so avoiding destroying bone or adjacent structures such as teeth or the inferior dental nerve. Marsupialisation is both a diagnostic and therapeutic procedure as it produces material for histological examination and removes the cystic pressure and stops further invasion of the cancellous bone. This technique is useful for large lesions in the maxilla, or where conventional enucleation would damage the inferior dental nerve or weaken the mandible and predispose it to fracture. Afterwards, the mucosa will try to heal over the hole, so normally the cyst cavity is packed to prevent this for at least two weeks. We prefer to use Whitehead's varnish on ribbon gauze to pack the cavity as it is antiseptic, and it sets firmly and prevents food from getting into the cavity. The pack is then removed by reducing it in stages so that healing takes place around it. Once the cavity is healed almost completely, we can carry out an enucleation for the final tissue, which should be near the surface.

Some rare non-odontogenic lesions such as ossifying fibroma, cemento-osseous dysplasia, and fibrous dysplasia can look cystic when they first start. If they are thought to be a cyst initially, then it doesn't matter as they are benign. They just have more careful

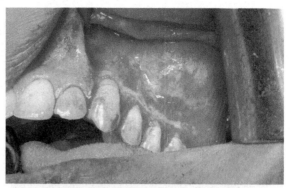
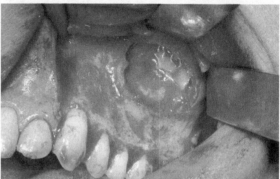
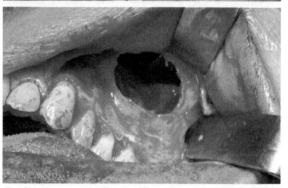

Radicular cyst of maxilla presented with bony expansion as seen top. Below: the cyst cavity exposed and cyst decompressed. Bottom: ready to sew up

---

Non-Odontogenic Cysts with Epithelial Lining

Nasopalatine Duct Cyst: formed from cells in vestigial nasopalatine duct; seen as midline radiolucency in palate; radiographically must be distinguished from normal nasopalatine duct i.e. more than 7 mms diameter

Nasolabial Cyst: rare; seen in soft tissue in nasolabial fold; formed from nasolabial duct cells

Sublingual Dermoid: Presents as swelling in floor of mouth; arises deep beneath tongue; arises from pharyngeal arch; has thick lining and contains thick keratin

---

Bone Cavity Cysts without Epithelial Lining

Solitary bone cyst (simple): usually in mandible in young people; frequently a chance radiographic finding; usually operated on for diagnosis; at operation there is no fluid or lining; healing occurs spontaneously

Aneurysmal Bone Cyst: rare cause of painless swelling; looks like a cyst on x-ray; curettage of the bloody cellular contents is curative but it can recur

34. <u>Introduction to Facial Skin Cancer</u>

Surgery for facial skin cancer has been increasingly carried out in OMFS departments in recent years. It was traditionally the work of plastic surgeons, who still do most of this work; however, there is plenty for everyone. Most of the patients are elderly and pleasant, the surgery is not taxing and most cases are very suitable for outpatient operations, carried out using local anaesthetic. We include this topic to help the core dental trainee understand the work of the speciality. Dental surgeons spend their practising careers looking at faces. Skin cancer is common, and it is a good thing for them to understand and be able to recognise the disease.

Incidence

Cancer of the skin (squamous and basal cell carcinoma and malignant melanoma), is responsible for about 20% of all new cancer cases reported in the UK but only a small proportion of the deaths. Malignant melanoma compromises about 10% of skin cancer cases but is responsible for most of the skin cancer deaths.

There has been an increasing incidence of skin cancer over the last few decades, the main culprit being ultra-violet radiation, mostly from sunlight, but also artificial. The other risk factors are increasing age, family history, multiple moles, fair skin which tends to burn easily on exposure to the sun, and immunosuppressants.

As with all cancers, treatment should be undertaken as part of a multidisciplinary team, which includes surgeons, an oncologist, pathologist, a clinical nurse specialist, and a dermatologist. The initial referral from the primary care physician should ideally be to the dermatologist who will be able, in most cases, to make a confident diagnosis clinically without histology; this is not the case with most other cancers. Often they will use a dermatoscope, which uses polarised light to

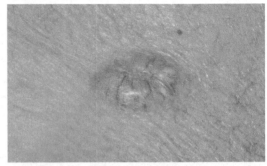

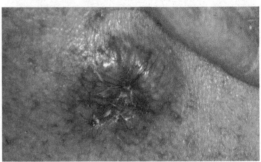

Basal Cell Carcinoma. Above are examples of the most common, nodular type. It is a pearly translucent papule or nodule with a central depression or crater, telangiectasia and a rolled waxy margin.

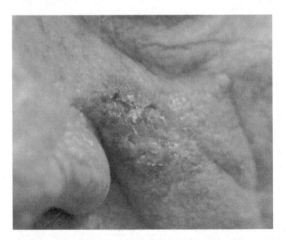

The least common morphoeic BCC is atrophic, white, slightly eroded or crusted plaque often looking like a scar. It is the most aggressive and difficult to treat as it is very difficult to define the margins. This lesion is very suitable for treatment with Mohs micrographic surgery or radiotherapy

---

<u>**Suspect malignant melanoma if:**</u>

A:- Asymmetrical
B:- Border irregular
C:- Colour not uniform
D:- Diameter more than 6 mms
E:- Evolving

---

produce a very clear image which is magnified and can be recorded.

Management options

Dermatologists often carry out curettage of small squamous and basal cells carcinomas, a technique not normally used by surgeons. The soft cancer is scraped out with a curette and requires some considerable experience to differentiate, by feel, the cancer tissue from normal skin. Pre-malignant lesions may be managed by freezing with liquid nitrogen spray or topical chemotherapy using 5-fluorouracil, diclofenac gel or imiquimod. Dermatologists may also carry out simple surgery of cases which require an elliptical incision with direct closure and refer only larger lesions which need flap repair or grafts; however, some dermatologists may do this surgery themselves.

Surgery

Most facial skin cancers can be excised with a simple elliptical incision and closed directly. The direction of 'Relaxed Skin Tension Lines' should be taken into account when planning the incision; the length of ellipse should be three times its width to ensure easy closure. Quite large lesions may be removed by this technique, particularly because most patients are elderly and have quite lax skin which can be undermined and therefore easily stretched. Larger wounds may be closed with transposition flaps of skin from an adjacent area or full thickness skin grafts, often taken from behind or in front of the ear or from the neck. Some wounds in areas difficult to close, such as the scalp, may be allowed to heal by secondary intention (as long as there is still periosteum covering the bone). Local flaps may be 'random pattern', where the blood supply depends on small randomly orientated subcutaneous blood vessels, or 'axial pattern', where the tissue is based on an artery. Here, the length can be much longer without compromising the perfusion of the tip.

Mohs micrographic surgery is a technique normally carried out by surgical dermatologists for larger malignant or pre-malignant lesions with a high risk of recurrence due to poorly defined margins, histological type, or location. Lesions in the central face around the eyes, nose or mouth generally have a poorer prognosis. In Mohs technique, the lesion is removed in stages, with a pathologist examining specimens from the periphery of the wound using frozen sections over several hours, or paraffin wax sections over several days. This approach is intensive in labour and hence expense, but has been shown to produce very high cure rates. Once the dermatologist and pathologist are

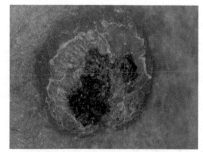

Squamous Cell Carcinoma. The lesion is hard with a rolled edge and ulcerated on the surface which has been bleeding

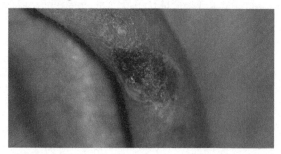

An early SSC lesion on the outer helix of the ear in sun-damaged skin

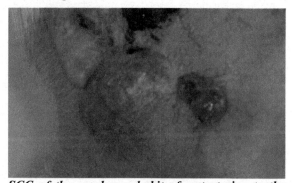

SCC of the ear has a habit of metastasing to the lymph nodes within the parotid many years later

Relaxed Skin Tension Lines

These correspond to orientation of collagen in dermis and are parallel to underlying muscle fibres.

Where possible surgical incisions should be made in the direction of the lines to produce better healing with less scarring.

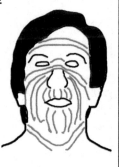

confident that all the lesion has been removed, the resulting defect can be referred for reconstructive surgery using soft tissue flaps.

Surgical treatment has the lowest overall failure rate for facial skin cancer. However, radiotherapy may be useful as an adjuvant treatment for larger squamous or recurrent multiple basal cell carcinomas; or it may be used as a primary treatment where a patient cannot tolerate surgery. Radiotherapy is generally less convenient, has the risk of radionecrosis and produces an inferior cosmetic result, although this is seldom an issue for older patients. Should a radiotherapy treated lesion recur, it cannot be used a second time and any subsequent surgery will be compromised by tissue damage and healing will be prolonged.

Malignant melanoma is radio resistant. Treatment should be primarily excising the lesion with a wide local margin after the case has been discussed by the skin cancer multidisciplinary team.

It is essential with all surgical procedures that all cancerous tissue is removed. Where the surgeon is not sure, the wound can be dressed and reconstructed at a later date or further tissue removed after the pathology specimen has been examined. The wound can later be skin grafted or left to heal by secondary intention.

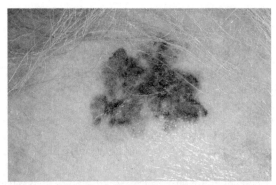

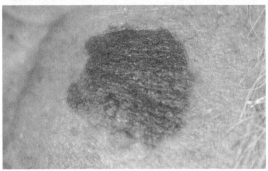

Malignant Melanoma. Above are examples of nodular malignant melanoma. They have irregular margins and pigmentation in varying shades of brown and black. The malignant cells grow up to form nodules and down to invade sub-dermal tissues, regional and distant lymph nodes and eventually liver, lungs and brain

---

Nomenclature

Papule: A circumscribed solid elevation of skin

Nodule: A palpable solid lesion in the skin or subcutaneous tissue, it extends deeper than a papule

Macule: A circumscribed flat area of discolouration without elevation or depression of surface

Plaque: A well-circumscribed, elevated, superficial, solid lesion, greater than 1 cm in diameter

Nevus: A circumscribed benign overgrowth of tissues which are normally present in the skin

In-situ: A lesion which contains malignant cells that have not metastasised or extended beyond the epidermis

Telangectasia: small dilated blood vessels visible near the surface

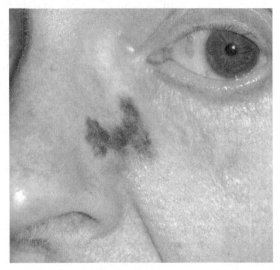

Superficial spreading melanoma grows horizontally rather than vertically down. It is macular or only slightly palpable

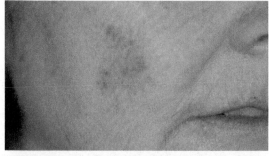

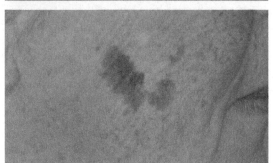

Lentigo Maligna, also known as Hutchinson's freckle. It is analogous to pre-malignant change in the oral mucosa, an 'in-situ' malignant melanoma; above are two examples. Note the varying colour. Biopsies from different parts of the lesion will show variable change so the lesions require complete removal often needing extensive surgery (for a lesion which might not become frankly invasive anyway)

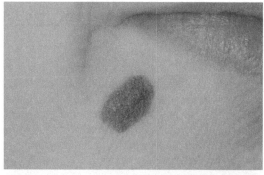

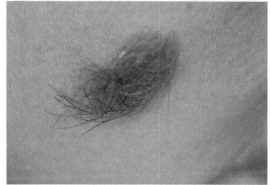

Melanocytic nevi are benign, and may be congenital or acquired. They vary greatly in appearance and may be flat, elevated, smooth, rough, sessile or polyp like. The symmetric shapes, regular borders, uniform colour and small size suggest these lesions are benign. The lower one is intradermal (it has hair). Bleeding or a change in size, colour or shape are suspicious of malignancy

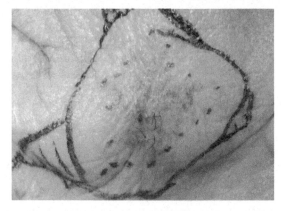

The black area within this facial lentigo maligna is nodular malignant melanoma arising. The dots mark the visible extent of the lesion and the continuous line the extent of the resection about to be undertaken

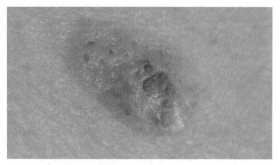

Seborrhoeic keratoses are benign, they mostly occur from middle age onwards so that most elderly people have some. Pigmentation is variable, some may be very dark and if flat may appear like a melanoma. No treatment is necessary

35. <u>Management of Temporomandibular Joint Pain and Dysfunction</u>

This chapter is about pain in the temporomandibular joint, the masticatory muscles and dysfunction of the joint associated with displacement of the joint disc and muscle spasm. We will not consider the rarer problems of disorders of growth or ankylosis of the joint which present to Oral and Maxillofacial Surgeons.

Anatomy and function

The temporomandibular joint is a synovial joint containing a fibrocartilage disc which divides it into two joint spaces. In the lower space, a rotation occurs between the head of the mandibular condyle and the disc. In the upper space, the disc translates forward from its neutral position within the glenoid fossa of the temporal bone down the sloping articular eminence. The masseter, temporalis and medial pterygoid muscles close the mouth and the lateral pterygoid pulls the head of the condyle and disc forward on closing. Maximum mouth opening requires both the rotation and forward translocation of the mandibular condyle. Should the forward movement of the head of the condyle be impeded, such as if the disc is displaced forward, then only the rotation will occur and mouth opening will be small.

Pain and dysfunction

Pain may occur in the joint alone, or the muscles alone, but is most commonly related to the joint and muscles together. This can be accompanied by clicking or crunching noises, locking (which may be intermittent or continuing) or deviation of the jaw on opening; these symptoms can occur with or without pain. The causation is not completely understood, but the latter (dysfunctional) symptoms are considered being related to forward and medial displacement of the joint disc and/or muscle spasm. Pain may be referred from one part of the masticatory apparatus to another and may affect one side or be bilateral.

About one third of people have symptoms at one time or another, but in many cases these are mild and transitory so that only a minority seeks professional advice or help. It may occur at any age, but it is predominantly from age 17 to 40 years and it is females who seek help most frequently.

Most cases appear to have no precipitating cause, but there is an association with 'parafunctional' habits such as clenching or grinding the teeth or chewing gum. There may also be an association with prolonged opening of the mouth for dental treatment, prolonged singing, playing musical instruments with the mouth, and recent trauma to the face. Emotions are thought to contribute, particularly stress, anxiety, depression, anger and hostility. Symptoms may fluctuate; locking seems to occur more frequently in the mornings, and in most cases, resolution is eventually spontaneous and complete. As with idiopathic facial pain, there is an association with chronic pains in other parts of the body, irritable bowel syndrome and chronic fatigue. Muscular pain may be related to fibromyalgia elsewhere in the body.

History and examination findings

A full history should be taken from the patient, which should include enquiry about pain, restriction of opening, locking, and joint noises. One should also ask if there is any other joint pathology or inflammatory arthropathy.

The examination should include palpation of the joint and lateral pterygoid, masseter and temporalis muscles to determine whether there is tenderness over the joint or muscles. Mouth opening is examined with observation of any deviation away from the midline. The gape should be measured between the upper and lower central incisors. This would normally be over 40 mm but will vary between individuals and especially is likely to be less in a class 2 division 2 incisor relationship. Its greater importance is for comparison, should the patient be seen on a subsequent occasion. It is also important to note the time of day as some patients report mouth opening to be most limited earlier in the mornings.

Disc position and symptoms

For most patients, an explanation of their symptoms can be made in terms of the position of the disc within the joint. In most cases, the disc will have displaced antero-medially and in these cases, the term 'internal derangement' of the joint is used. The disc is displaced 'with reduction' if it is partly displaced forward. When the condyle is translated forward, it resumes the same relationship to the disc that it would normally occupy in the closed position in the glenoid fossa. This can explain a 'click', which probably occurs when the head of the condyle moves forward over the thicker posterior band of the disc. The condylar head resumes its usual relationship to the disc. A click usually occurs on opening; it can occur on opening and closing (reciprocal click) but only rarely just on closing.

The disc is said to be displaced 'without reduction' if it is displaced so far forward and is bunched up in front of the condyle and remains in front of it in maximal opening. This may lead to the condyle being unable to move forward enough for the mouth to open completely or locked closed. Sometimes the mandible may open but will deviate towards the affected side because the condyle is prevented from translating forwards.

Around 30% of the population have a click and this in itself does not warrant treatment, nor does it imply the presence or predispose to the development of arthritis. In fact, the term arthritis of the TMJ should not be used other than reassurance that it is unlikely to occur.

However, these explanations are probably a simplification of what may be happening. The definitive way to visualise the position of the disc is with arthroscopy. MRI scans can visualise the position of the disc. They show that many people have displaced discs with no symptoms or signs at all. Symptoms may be due to muscle spasm alone. In the majority of cases, we do not request MRI scans; we believe that when the disc is anteriorly displaced with reduction, we can

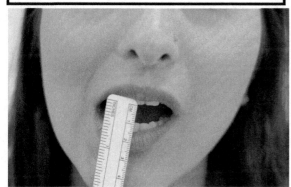

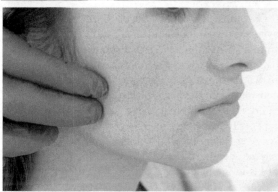

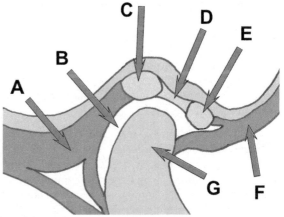

Diagram of position of disc in relation to condyle with mouth closed. A: Bilaminar zone, upper layer is elastic and lower is dense B: Lower joint space C: Thick posterior band D: Thin intermediate zone E: Anterior band F: Lateral pterygoid muscle inserted into the meniscus superiorly and the anterior of the condyle below G: Head of condyle.
The condyle moves forward more than the disc on opening

Top: Examination should include measurement of opening between the central incisors and any deviation on opening. Here the gape is limited to 9mms interincisal distance and the mandible is deviated to the right consequent upon disc displacement in the right joint.
Bottom: The masticatory muscles should be palpated to elicit any tenderness

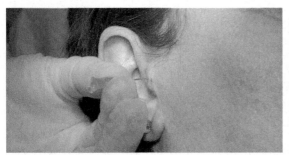

Arthrocentesis local anaesthesia: A topical anaesthetic is placed followed by a painless injection with dental Wand™, an 21 gauge needle is placed into the upper joint space and saline injected, pressure is felt when it is the correct place and a flashback of saline occurs. A second needle can now be placed and the joint space thoroughly irrigated with saline

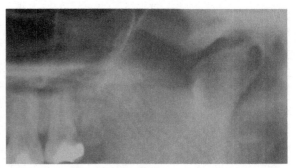

Arthrosis of the TMJ. This detail of an OPG image showed marked resorption of the head of the mandibular condyle. This was a chance finding on a routine image. The patient had no symptoms.

diagnose this reasonably accurately from the clinical history and examination alone, particularly the clicking. However, a disc which is anteriorly displaced without reduction is more difficult to predict. Sometimes there may be no symptoms or signs at all; in many, there will be just limitation of opening and deviation to the affected side.

Crepitus or grating may be due to degeneration of the disc, which may be worn, atrophic and/or torn; this may be accompanied by resorption of the head of the mandibular condyle. We associate crepitus from any joint with arthrosis or arthritis; however MRI scans have shown that a very deformed disc (round or folded) which is anteriorly displaced without reduction may lead to crepitus with no sign of bony degeneration in the condylar head, although this may come later. This may be particularly associated with tenderness of the lateral pterygoid muscles.

Condylar resorption may be seen on an orthopantomograph x-ray image, but we know that many joints which show evidence of quite severe degeneration on imaging produce no symptoms at all. You may see orthopantomograph images showing flattening of the head of the mandibular condyle, which are asymptomatic; here, it might be that the bone has remodelled in response to some former insult or it may be related to the plane of the tomographic cut.

We use the term 'internal derangement' to describe the condition where there are signs or symptoms of disc displacement and 'facial arthro-myalgia' where there is pain in the joint and/or the master and temporalis muscles but no signs or symptoms of disc displacement (other than pain).

Once a full history has been taken, and an examination made, imaging should be considered. There will almost always be a policy within the department you work in. Many would recommend an orthopantomograph which will complement clinical examination and aid diagnosis of any dental or bony oral pathology which might cause referred pain. It may reassure the patient that they have received a comprehensive assessment. To image the disc, an MRI scan may be used. However, we only use this if open surgery to the joint is contemplated as otherwise it will not have any bearing on the clinical management. In those, increasingly fewer, occasions when open surgery is considered, an MRI scan may be used to confirm the disc displacement for medico-legal reasons.

Prognosis

In most cases of internal derangement, the symptoms settle spontaneously with no intervention from us. Unfortunately, it is difficult to predict which patients' symptoms will not resolve. Our experience is that those who have symptoms of pain in the joint and masticatory muscles with no sign or history of internal derangement have a poorer prognosis, especially if accompanied by chronic pain elsewhere. Another category who do less well are those with internal derangement symptoms following some sort of facial trauma, often a whiplash or similar injury.

Conservative management

So our initial management for most cases will be to explain and carry out no active treatment. We advise patients to limit their mouth opening by stifling yawns, avoiding dental treatment until it has all settled, to have a soft diet and take care to chew evenly on both sides and to avoid chewing gum or any other habits which might put an unnecessary strain on the masticatory apparatus.

There are numerous management strategies that have been used and for which benefit has been claimed. However, we believe that the balance of informed opinion is against any irreversible treatment which is potentially damaging, such as occlusal adjustment and mandibular repositioning appliances with orthodontics. Some departments may use bite splints and we believe that there is some weak evidence that they may help with pain, but we do not use them as a primary care dentist can provide them.

Capsaicin or non-steroidal anti-inflammatory medication may be useful if applied topically for pain and a low dose of tricyclic medication for longer term muscular pain. Some patients may present with a 'closed lock', which is assumed to be because of anterior displacement of the discs 'without reduction'. Spasm of the masticatory muscles contributes to a closed lock and a low dose of diazepam, for a maximum of two weeks, may be prescribed in the anticipation that it will help with the muscular problem and facilitate a quicker recovery. Arthrocentesis has been shown to be of benefit where an acute severe restriction of opening occurs. Injection of the masticatory muscles with botulinum toxin has also been reported to be helpful for refractory muscular pain and some prescribe physiotherapy but we are unconvinced that this had any long-term benefit.

Although most patients eventually recover, this is not always the case. Formerly, surgery was often used to correct the problem, usually an open operation to free up the disc from its anterior displacement and suture it back into position. If severely damaged, the disc may be removed. This operation may be helpful, but there is also evidence that disc plication alone is not a satisfactory long-term treatment, as the disc displacement may recur. Surgery should always be considered with some apprehension, as once the disc is operated on or removed, the joint will never be normal again.

Surgery may allow a patient to once again open their mouth without pain, but they are often left with a permanent deviation of the mandible on opening, which generally does not concern them. However, there is always a greater risk of joint degeneration once it has been opened. A patient who has been operated on for relief of pain may find that pain continues after the surgery (following a brief placebo response) and the pain then becomes intractable. In this case, the surgeon

Possible Non Surgical Treatments
Bite splints
Physiotherapy
Ultrasound
Acupuncture
Soft laser treatment
Massage
Cognitive behaviour therapy

may be blamed for the pain and further surgery demanded.

A less invasive surgical approach is arthroscopy, where the upper joint space is visualised through a scope; this is the definitive way of making an accurate diagnosis. It is possible to suture the disc through an arthroscope but usually just an attempt is made to free the disc by simply breaking up adhesions and washing the upper joint space out. This is normally carried out under general anaesthetic.

An alternative is arthrocentesis and in our hands, we have found this simpler technique to be equally effective in helping recovery, although it does not produce an instant cure. Two needles are placed into the upper joint space and lavage is carried out with saline. This can be done with general or local anaesthetic; our audit has shown better results with local anaesthetic in the dental chair, although others have found the opposite. Some surgeons have published that improvement in symptoms is as good with arthrocentesis as the more invasive arthroscopy. It has also been reported that the instillation of morphine during the procedure is helpful for pain control. Patients should be warned that improvement in symptoms is the goal and they should not expect an immediate cure, but that complete resolution is usual in most (but not all) cases, sometime later. They should also be informed that joint noises may not be relieved or may return, but that these alone are not important.

36. <u>Introduction to Chronic Facial Pain</u>

Oral and Maxillofacial Surgery departments will all receive a continuous supply of patients suffering from chronic pain who will want a cure. As surgeons we are not the appropriate people for management of chronic conditions which do not benefit from surgery but in the case of facial pain, we may be well suited to investigate and diagnose before discharging the patient back to the primary care doctor or dentist with an explanation of symptoms and advice where further help might be found.

Chronic pain specialists have superior experience in use of the medications as well as teams containing psychologists, councillors and physiotherapist and techniques such as acupuncture, cognitive behavioural therapy and transcutaneous nerve stimulation.

History and examination

We always start with a detailed history of the pain and other pains the patient has experienced. In idiopathic chronic facial pain, the patient will probably have or have had chronic pains in other parts of the body or face, and these must be elicited. Many patients with chronic pain may have certain personality traits, which may have exacerbated the pain. A full examination must include a detailed dental examination, as our experience has been that sometimes busy dentists can miss dental disease, which is not blindingly obvious. This will obviously include imaging. It is often said that the diagnosis of much chronic facial pain is one of exclusion, but in practice a patient with a history of over three months of pain is unlikely to have a peripherally organic lesion or disease process which is amenable to surgery.

Once a diagnosis has been made, a detailed explanation must be given. This must be reinforced by a summary in writing, which is often best made as a letter to the patient with a copy to the primary care clinician who referred them. We always reassure the patient that they do not have cancer and this is easier for them to accept if they have received an MRI or CT scan of the facial area.

Most people's experience of pain will be of acute pain. The difference between acute and chronic pain must be explained, an acute pain being physiological and useful because it warns the body of damage and allows evasive action to be taken, whereas chronic pain is pathological, abnormal and dysfunctional and has no useful purpose. Once a chronic pain syndrome has developed, elimination can be very much more difficult and coping may be a more realistic goal.

Pain perception

The perception of pain is a complicated biochemical, structural and physiological mechanism involving local chemical mediators of pain, peripheral nervous transmission and central perception. These are modified by downward inhibitory neural mediation in which mood, personality and emotion take a part. In many cases peripheral lesions or disease processes which might be expected to lead to pain produce none; this confirms that the mechanism depends on factors beyond simple structural tissue damage.

The term 'chronic pain syndrome' suggests that the patient is suffering from a global entity; it is often associated with poor general health. Chronic pain may result from an injury which has modified the peripheral or central nervous system, leading to maladaptive processing of sensory information. This might be a particularly severe or poorly controlled episode of acute pain following an injury or even surgery. The effective management of acute pain may have a role in preventing some chronic pain. This 'neuropathic' pain is really a spectrum of disorders and may be idiopathic but may also occur as a result of specific infection such as varicella zoster as in the condition post herpetic neuralgia.

The chronic pain syndromes

We will now discuss the common chronic pain syndromes that you are likely to meet but will leave pain related to the temporomandibular joint and masticatory muscle considered in another chapter.

<u>Trigeminal neuralgia</u> occurs mostly, but not exclusively, in the elderly. Diagnosis is from the clinical history and normally consists of sharp shooting pains each lasting for a few seconds several times each day. They are typically initiated by light touching of the face and mostly the 2nd and 3rd divisions of the trigeminal nerve are affected, usually unilateral. Classically, the pain may be started by shaving or brushing teeth, causing the patient to cease these activities. Remissions of the pain can occur and last for weeks or even months before it returns. The usual management of this particularly severe pain is with the anticonvulsant carbamazepine which is used for the severe shooting pain and tricyclic antidepressants, which may help with background pain.

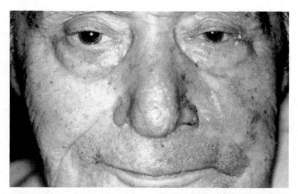

Herpes zoster reactivated in patient immunocompromised by chemotherapy for malignant disease. The vesicles within the erythema are just healing but the severe pain lasted for many months and was only partly helped by gabapentin and amitriptyline

Carbamazepine should be started on a low dose and blood counts monitored as it can lead to marrow suppression, hepatic and renal function are tested initially. The medication induces enzymes in the liver, where it is metabolised, so with time, increased doses are needed to effect the same improvement. Drowsiness, ataxia and nausea are associated with the medication. If this occurs, it may be prudent to change the medication to oxcarbazepine. All patients should have an MR scan of the floor of the middle cranial fossa and a consultation with a neurosurgeon because trigeminal neuralgia can be caused by compression of the root of the trigeminal nerve by vessels so surgery to decompress it (microvascular decompression) can effect a cure. For those who are unfit for open surgery, stereotactic radiosurgery, with a gamma knife, can also cure it. Patients with multiple sclerosis are more frequently affected and at a younger age; for them, the condition tends to be more severe and intractable.

Post herpetic neuralgia is a facial pain caused by reactivation of the varicella-zoster virus which has remained dormant in the trigeminal nucleus after the initial exposure as chickenpox. There are eruptions of vesicles often accompanied by erythema. Severe pain can result and often last for months or years after the vesicles have healed. This is primarily a disease of the immunocompromised or elderly. The pain can resolve after months, but in the meantime it is incapacitating. Management can be with topical capsaicin administered as a low dose cream or higher dose patch, topical lidocaine, gabapentin and tricyclic antidepressants.

Persistent idiopathic facial pain is a term introduced in recent years which encompassed the previous diagnoses of atypical facial pain and atypical odontalgia. It is a diagnosis of exclusion as it is made on the clinical history and absence of any pathology found on examination of the mouth and face. However, the symptoms described are usually indicative of the diagnosis soon after the consultation begins.

The terms atypical facial pain and atypical odontalgia are still in widespread use because they describe two clinical syndromes with different prognoses. Atypical facial pain is not a very specific pain. It is usually experienced in the mid-face, can occur bilaterally, is deep-seated and poorly localised. The sufferer is usually a middle-aged female and often gives a history of chronic pain elsewhere in the body at different times. In addition, they may have suffered from irritable bowel syndrome and chronic fatigue.

The mainstay of our management is to reassure the patient of the absence of cancer, advise them of the nature of chronic and neuropathic pain and how their condition might be helped whilst acknowledging that this is not an expertise of our speciality. Tricyclic antidepressant medication has been shown to be helpful, but it is important to explain to the patient that this is independent of its use for depression. A dose lower than that used for depression is used and it is important to explain that any beneficial effect will take two or three weeks to appear but that side effects, particularly drowsiness, come on immediately but often decrease later. Serotonin and norepinephrine re-uptake inhibitors may also help and cause fewer side effects;

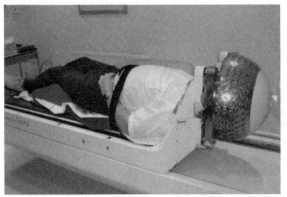

Patient with trigeminal neuralgia receiving stereotactic radiosurgery in neurosurgery centre with a gamma knife. His pain was helped by carbamazepine but the gamma knife cured it. However more patients will have microvascular decompression which is more reliable

selective serotonin re-uptake inhibitors tend not to help. The patient should be discharged with this advice and told that after a few weeks, the primary care physician will probably need to adjust the medication to achieve the optimal outcome.

The key to success is compliance and insight into the nature of the problem. It is possible to completely wreck this by repeated unnecessary and repetitive investigations or physical treatment. The patient should

therefore be seen only by a mature, confident, and experienced clinician.

Less common, atypical odontalgia occurs in the teeth and alveolus. The patient often presents having had multiple dental procedure often culminating in extraction, each leading to a brisk placebo response followed by a return of the pain in adjacent teeth or the area of extraction. Here insight into the problem is very difficult to achieve, and it is not unusual for a single patient to be seen by multiple dentists each contributing unnecessary treatment. In atypical odontalgia, the prognosis is significantly worse than atypical facial pain. In atypical facial pain, the prognosis is worse when the patient is a male. It is possible for patients to see a chronic pain specialist, but we have seen little evidence of them being able to help.

Medication	Use	Side effects	Our comment
Tricyclic antidepressants	Neuropathic pain particularly atypical facial pain, post herpetic neuralgia	Dry mouth, drowsiness initially, blurred vision, constipation, weight gain or loss, postural hypotension	Lower dose than for depression, benefit delayed for 2 or 3 weeks then dose needs titrating
Serotonin norepinephrine re-uptake inhibitor (antidepressants)	As above	Nausea, drowsiness, loss of appetite, weight, and sleep, dizziness, fatigue, headache, diminished libido, anxiety, pulse and blood pressure	Nausea tends to settle, less sedating than tricyclics
Carbamazepine (anti-convulsant)	Neuropathic pain best for trigeminal neuralgia	Suppression of white blood cells and platelets monitor blood counts periodically	Causes liver induction so increasing dose needed with time. Monitor liver function before treatment
Gabapentin (anticonvulsant)	Neuropathic pain particularly post herpetic neuralgia	Dizziness, drowsiness, peripheral oedema, and gait disturbance	
Pregbalin (anticonvulsant)	neuropathic pain particularly post herpetic neuralgia	Drowsiness, dizziness effect on cognition and co-ordination	Use if other treatments have failed

Medications used for chronic facial pain

37. <u>Understanding Potentially Malignant Oral Disorders</u>

A vast number of patients each year will be referred to Oral and Maxillofacial departments because they have lesions in the mouth which are potentially malignant. These are erythroplakia (which are red patches which are often dysplastic, and a high risk for malignancy), leukoplakia (which are white and approximately 30% may become malignant), mixed red and white lesions, oral sub-mucous fibrosis and lichen planus (which has the potential to become malignant but has a very low transformation rate). Overall, the prevalence of these lesions may be between 0.2 to 11 %, depending on which study is the most accurate. They have been reported as having an overall rate of transformation to cancer of between 1 and 30%.

These lesions represent a challenge because they are large in number and the majority will never become malignant. We need to decide which of these should be followed up and if there is any intervention, we can make which will improve the prognosis of those that will.

History

In most cases, a clinical diagnosis may be made after taking a full clinical and medical history combined with clinical examination. The history should always include a full medical, medication, allergy history as well as enquiry about smoking, drinking and chewing habits and presence of skin lesions. Examination should include palpation for cervical lymph nodes and examination of all the oral mucosa with a good light. The lesions should be palpated with a gloved finger and a note made of oral hygiene and any sharp or uneven teeth or prostheses.

Some white patches (or ulcers) on the buccal mucosa or tongue may be frictional from sharp or broken teeth. Removal of the cause will allow resolution of the problem but be aware that sharp teeth can rub cancers too. Careful follow up or immediate biopsy of the lesion is essential to be reassured of a benign diagnosis.

Lichen Planus Types of Lesion
Reticular Plaques Atrophic Erosive Desquamative gingivitis

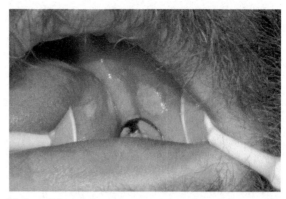

Lichenoid reactions can occur to dental restorative material composites, gold, cobalt or most commonly amalgam as here. This may be a sensitivity to amalgam but patch testing is generally unhelpful. Removing the filling and replacement with an alternative material is often rewarded with a resolution or improvement of the lesion but is not guaranteed

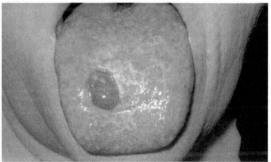

A florid lichen planus of the tongue with a granulation in an erosion

Lichen planus

Most white patches in the mouth will be oral lichen planus, a chronic cell-mediated immune condition of unknown cause leading to hyperkeratosis. It occurs mostly in females of late middle age. Most cases will be asymptomatic and no treatment is necessary or possible. The clinical issue, particularly for the plaque like patches, is which ones to biopsy to exclude dysplasia or malignancy or to confirm the diagnosis. The typical histological appearance is of lymphocytic infiltration into the superficial connective tissue and liquefaction degeneration of the basal cells. Lichen planus does not contain evidence of dysplasia. The term 'lichenoid dysplasia' is used when a dysplastic lesion is accompanied by a dense lymphocytic response is seen in the sub-epithelial connective tissue layer like lichen planus.

Except with betel quid chewers (betel leaf, tobacco, slaked lime and areca nut) there is a low incidence of malignancy in the buccal mucosa. We believe that in the very common circumstance of obvious reticular lichen planus at this site, the patient may be reassured of the diagnosis without biopsy and no follow up arranged. The patient should be advised to return if symptoms occur or there is a change in appearance. For plaque-like and ulcerative lesions, a biopsy will be necessary to make a diagnosis. If lichen planus is diagnosed, follow up for a couple of years may be prudent, with further review by the primary care doctor or dentist after that. There is, however, no evidence that this will be effective in either early diagnosis or of survival from a possible squamous cancer.

Leukoplakia

Leukoplakia is a clinical diagnosis made for a white patch which cannot be wiped off, and for which another diagnosis which has not increased risk of cancer has been excluded. Thus an acute pseudomembranous candidiasis will be excluded as it can be wiped off. A white spongy naevus, frictional keratosis, habitual lip and cheek biting, chemical burn, leukoedema, lichen planus, lichenoid reaction, hairy leucoplakia, smoker's keratosis of the palate and skin grafts all have a separate diagnosis.

It is probable that the risk of malignant change is greater in lesions which are large, cover several oral mucosal surfaces, are situated on the floor of the mouth or ventral surface of the tongue. Those that are infected with candida hyphae are thick and non-homogeneous (rather than thin and uniform) and particularly if they are speckled containing red areas are also of higher risk. Proliferative verrucous leucoplakia with multiple foci and covering a wide area is considered the worst clinical appearance for malignant change. Risk factors for developing a potentially malignant leukoplakia are tobacco, alcohol and betel quid chewing. The risk of malignant transformation may be greater in older females and if the patient has extensive lesions not associated with smoking and high alcohol intake.

Dysplasia

These lesions should always be investigated with a biopsy. The presence of dysplasia is a prognostic indicator of potential malignant change. Dysplasia is graded as mild, moderate or severe, but the grading is inexact with much inter- and intra-observer variation. A mild dysplasia can be reversed if a patient with a smoking or alcohol habit can be persuaded to stop, but not necessarily. For severe dysplasias, surgical excision, often with a carbon dioxide laser, is frequently carried out. This is considered to reduce the incidence of, or delay, malignant change. It is not carried out for mild dysplasia, and for moderate dysplasia, it may not be beneficial. For very large lesions, excision can be a formidable problem. The alternative is to carefully observe the lesions as malignant change is far from inevitable. Leucoplakia is probably not homogenous histologically and one part of the lesion may have mild or moderate dysplasia and another part may have a micro-invasive carcinoma or carcinoma-in-situ (cancer that does not extend beyond the epithelium). Techniques such as staining with toluidine blue, cytology with a brush biopsy and optical techniques are alleged to predict dysplasia, but we believe these are yet to be fully evaluated. There is evidence that staining with Lugol's iodine before laser excision of dysplasia may show up dysplasia beyond the visible margin. This may facilitate wider excision, which in turn will decrease recurrence of the lesion and malignant transformation.

Where possible, removal of the entire lesion with a carbon dioxide laser will allow histological examination of all the lesion. If dysplasia is present may prevent malignant change in (possibly) half of cases but not all. Long term follow up is essential. However, many patients will be quite elderly and may not tolerate multiple laser excisions, especially as it is

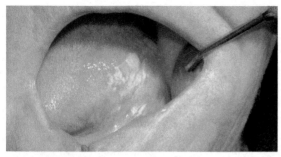

Dysplasic lesion on the side of the tongue. The tongue should always be regarded with suspicion. Removal of the lesion with CO_2 will allow all the lesion to be analysed by the pathologist (in case it contains a small, micro-invasive cancer or carcinoma-in-situ) but will not necessarily reduce the risk of malignant change. Careful advice and follow up is desirable.

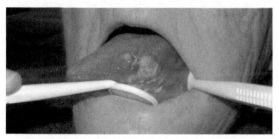

The same patient 3 years later; a cancer has arisen in the lesion. The sutures are from the biopsy

not certain they will get a malignancy and surgery does not guarantee that they will not.

Erythroplakia

Erythroplakia, or red patch, is a less common but sinister potentially malignant lesion; it is often mixed with white speckles or areas.

Sub-mucous fibrosis

Sub-mucous fibrosis occurs predominantly in Asians and is caused by chewing the areca nut. It is very common worldwide but not necessarily within the UK. Patients will experience burning of the mucosa and sensitivity to spicy foods. The mucosa has a blanched appearance, and an increased risk of malignant transformation. Fibrous bands form beneath the mucosa, leading to progressive decrease in mouth opening. Sub-mucous fibrosis is very challenging for the clinician, not only attempting to help with the progressive trismus but monitoring the oral mucosa for malignant change when mouth opening is inadequate.

In conclusion, the management of potentially malignant conditions of the oral mucosa is awkward because they may be mimicked by many lesions without malignant potential. They are often not homogenous; most of them do not become malignant and there is no universally agreed management strategy. Management of each lesion must be dictated by an experienced clinician and not delegated to trainees.

In our experience, most mistakes in management we have seen have been related to lesions on the lateral border of the tongue, which were not taken seriously enough. An apparently small area of mucosal damage caused by dental trauma can be mimicked by invasive cancer. Dental trauma must be observed to heal completely (not just improved) after removal of the apparent cause before a patient may be reassured and discharged from follow up. A small tongue cancer can behave aggressively, but if diagnosed, early treatment may be curative.

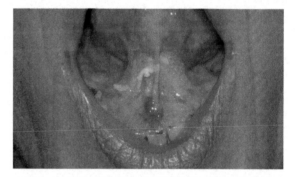

Floor of mouth keratosis has a high potential for malignant transformation.

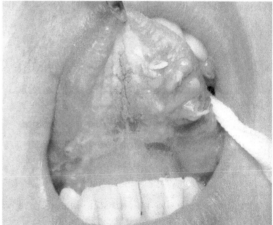

Field change. The patient has widespread dysplasia around the mouth which produced multiple metachronous tumours. Very difficult to deal with. The sutures are from a recent biopsy

38. Oral Candidiasis

Patients may be referred with symptoms or signs related to oral candidiasis or it may present associated with some other problem for which they are being seen. About half of the population will have the main organism, the fungus Candida Albicans living within their mouths as a commensal, but in certain circumstances it may overgrow and become an 'opportunistic' infection. Below, we have listed some of the commonest opportunities candida may have to overgrow.

Angular cheilitis

This is probably the most common presentation. It is an atrophic erythematous area at the oral commissure. It can be associated with any cause of oral candida and the characteristic appearance normally does not require any special investigation. The intra oral problem should be dealt with primarily and the angular cheilitis may be treated with topical miconazole gel. However, you should know angular cheilitis may be caused by staph aureus from the nose or this organism may co-exist with candida in the lesions. If there is no clear association with intra oral infection, then a swab to diagnose candida or staphylococcus may be useful.

Chronic atrophic candidiasis

Angular cheilitis is most commonly associated with chronic atrophic candidiasis - denture stomatitis, also called denture sore mouth, which is usually not sore. Most commonly, the patient is a full denture wearer with old and worn dentures. This leads to a reduced vertical dimension so that the folds of the oral commissure are deeper. This mechanical problem predisposes to the infective one. There is an atrophic area beneath the fitting surface of the upper denture, often the patient wears the dentures at night. The

---

Oral Candidiasis - Some Precipitating factors

Alteration of the oral environment - dentures

Change in oral flora - antibiotics

Compromised immunity from disease - diabetes, haematological malignancy, HIV

Immunosuppressive medication - chemotherapy for malignancy, steroids for acute or chronic disease

Dry mouth - caused by many medications, radiotherapy for oral cancer

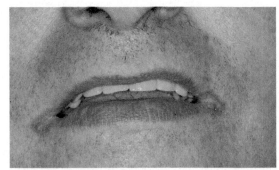

A typical angular chelitis. The white areas in the commissures suggest it has been present a long time

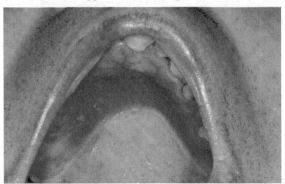

Same patient. There is a severe denture stomatitis beneath the old acrylic partial denture. This is severe with a rough appearance to the erythematous denture bearing area. The recommended management was: remove dentures at night and soak in half strength Milton, amphotericin lozenges sucked slowly x3 daily with dentures out and because it was severe miconazole gel applied to the denture fitting area and oral commissures. Then we referred to a dentist for attention to her decayed teeth and a for a new denture

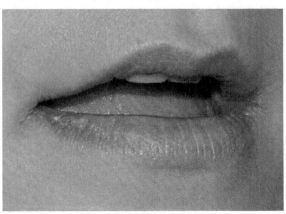

A young woman with angular chelitis, she had no sign of oral candidiasis. Swabs were taken from the commissures and her nose which revealed the cause was staphylococcus aureus from her nose

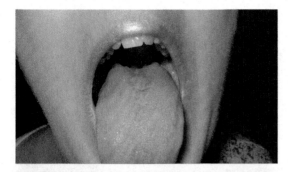

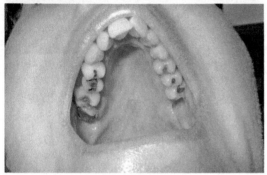

Above: median rhomboid glossitis in a young woman. Below: 'kissing' lesion on palate. These were treated with topical antifungals, the palatal lesion disappeared but the tongue lesion persisted. No biopsy was carried out

problem can usually be dealt with by requesting the patient to leave their dentures out at night and soaked in a half strength solution of Milton (hypochlorite). When the clinical evidence of infection has subsided, new dentures can be made with a slightly increased vertical dimension. This may be supplemented with amphotericin lozenges sucked three times daily while the dentures are soaking in Milton. Miconazole gel can be applied to the fitting surface of the upper denture.

Acute atrophic candidiasis

This may present as a soreness or bad taste in the mouth and may be related to antibiotic use (particularly if broad spectrum) and again may be asymptomatic. It may be seen as an erythematous area or a depapillated area of the tongue. Where the tongue is involved, look for a 'kissing' lesion on the palate where one area has 'infected' the other. Again, the problem may well settle on its own once antibiotics have been stopped, if indeed this is the cause. Otherwise nystatin suspension, amphotericin lozenges or miconazole gel may help or fluconazole systemically if severe.

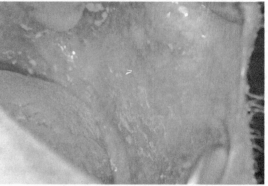

Acute pseudomembranous candidiasis (thrush) on the buccal mucosa. Patient was asthmatic and was being treated for an acute chest infection with antibiotics and systemic steroid for exacerbation of the asthma. Although it would have cleared up when these medications stopped we treated it with fluconazole as it was sore and affecting the oropharynx as well

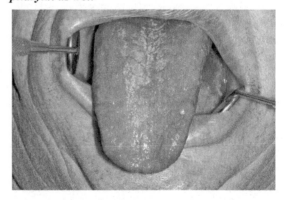

Acute pseudomembranous candidiasis on the tongue; it wiped off with a gauze swab and there were flecks of candida on the buccal mucosa similar to the image above

Median rhomboid glossitis

We do not know the cause of median rhomboid glossitis. It is usually asymptomatic and the patient may present because they are alarmed at the appearance and want a diagnosis. This is frequently associated with candidal infection and whereas antifungal medication may remove the candida, the lesion usually persists. A decision whether to biopsy the area needs to be made as it may represent a tumour. However, this is a site which is rarely involved with cancer, so a long history of the lesion being present, with no increase in size, would steer us into the decision not to biopsy.

Pseudomembranous candidiasis

Is commonly called thrush. It may have the appearance of white plaques or flecks on an inflamed mucosa. It may occur in babies but the primary care or paediatric doctor or nurse will not need our help with this. So we are likely to see it only in adults who may present with soreness, burning or a bad taste.

The diagnosis can be made from the history and the appearance. The white lesions may be wiped off the erythematous mucosa by holding the part steady in a swab and wiping with another gauze swab. Special tests are unlikely to be needed for diagnosis but a microbiological swab sample will cultivate the candida hyphae, which may be seen with haematoxylin & eosin staining or, more reliably, with periodic acid Schiff staining. As in all cases, there must be a reason for the candida growth and most frequently we have found this to be in patients with chronic obstructive pulmonary disease who have suffered an acute exacerbation secondary to an acute chest infection; the cause is usually their prescribed systemic steroids, inhaled steroids or broad-spectrum antibiotics. The oral problem normally resolves once their additional medication has ceased, but in the meantime, management may be with topical nystatin suspension or amphotericin lozenges or in severe cases systemic fluconazole.

Chronic hyperplasic candidiasis

Or candidal leukoplakia; it is really a leukoplakia which is infected with candida hyphae. The interesting question is whether the leukoplakia has been caused by the candida or it has just been secondarily infected by it. We do not know the answer to that question, but we can make two observations. Firstly, the lesions we have seen are usually on the buccal mucosa just within the oral commissure and secondly that in our

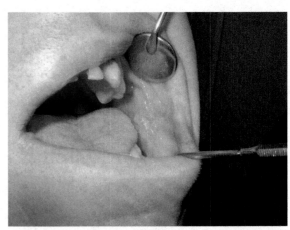

Chronic hyperplastic candidiasis just within the oral commissures. It would not wipe off with a gauze swab nor did it resolve with antifungal treatment

experience treating them with antifungals does not seem to get rid of the lesions.

The lesions will not wipe off with a gauze swab, so we start with a biopsy, which will show the leukoplakia to contain candida hyphae. Then we treat with a topical antifungal such as miconazole gel. We know leukoplakia is at greater risk of malignant transformation if infected with candida, so we tend to photograph them, completely excise the lesion with a carbon dioxide laser and then keep them under review.

Chronic mucocutaneous candidiasis

You are unlikely to see this is it does not present to oral and maxillofacial surgeons. It has a variety of systemic causes for reduced immunity to candida and presents in childhood with candida involvement of skin and all mucosal surfaces.

Occasionally you will see a patient with signs and/or symptoms of oral candidiasis with no obvious predisposing factors being present. In this case, we should always consider undiagnosed reasons for compromised immunity such as undiagnosed diabetes and be aware that there is a significantly higher risk of oral candidiasis in those infected with HIV.

39. <u>Ulcers and Bullae</u>

There are many causes of oral ulcers, vesicles and bullae. We will attempt to guide you on the principles and management of these lesions that you are likely to see in an oral and maxillofacial surgery department. We have listed the commonest and the less common lesions that you might see and which you should remember when assessing patients. For a comprehensive account of the rarer causes you should refer to specialist text of oral medicine.

A bulla is a fluid-filled cavity beneath or within the mucosa; the term vesicle is used if it is small (less than 5 mm across) and the lay term is a blister. A bulla in the mouth is likely to burst and present as an ulcer which is a break in the epithelium, you are therefore unlikely to see many bullae. The best chance of seeing an intact one is in <u>angina bullosa heamorrhagica,</u> which is commonly known as a blood blister. These are harmless but can be recurrent but usually they resolve completely.

Cancerous ulcer

The classical appearance of a <u>cancerous ulcer</u> is of induration with a raised rolled border. The ulcer is painless when small but becomes painful as it enlarges and invades neural tissue or becomes secondarily infected; a larger infected, cancerous ulcer of the mouth will have a characteristic smell. However, we have known cancers to mimic many other oral lesions and some cancers primarily infiltrate the tissues when small, causing minimal ulceration initially.

A suspected cancer or undiagnosed ulcer should be subjected to urgent biopsy, i.e. on the day they present to the clinic. It is important to remember a biopsy report which shows no evidence of cancer might do so because the specimen was too small, taken from an unrepresentative area or was difficult to interpret because of associated traumatic changes or secondary infection. No patient should be discharged from care with an undiagnosed ulcer. The author's record is three biopsies of an oral ulcer before the cancer that the patient feared and the clinician suspected was confirmed by histology.

Traumatic ulcers

These are fairly common in the mouth; they are usually very painful. Causes include prostheses, orthodontic appliances, sharp teeth and broken restorations. It is not uncommon for patients to present with ulcers on the side of the tongue related to prominent molar cusps which do not appear to be

---

> ### *Oral Ulcers - Most Important*
> **Cancer**
>
> ### *Oral Ulcers - Commonest*
> **Traumatic**
> **Erosive Lichen Planus**
> **Aphthae**
>
> ### *Oral Ulcers & Bullae - Less Common*
> **Primary Herpetic Gingivo Stomatitis**
> **Angina Bullosa Heamorrhagica**
> **Medication induced**
> **Acute Ulcerative Gingivitis**
> **Erythema Multiforme**
> **Benign Tumour**
> **Mucous Membrane Pemphigoid**
> **Pemphigus Vulgaris**
>
> *This list is not complete a specialist Oral Medicine text will include the rare causes of ulceration you are unlikely to see*

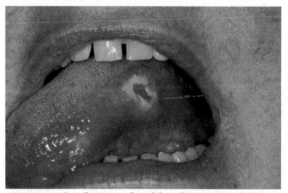

A traumatic ulcer on the side of a tongue. It is very painful. The diagnosis is suggested by the pain, the frictional keratosis around it's margin and the sharp tooth cusp you cannot see. We removed the cause and it was completely healed in two weeks. Many would biopsy this on the first attendance to exclude cancer. We think this is quite reasonable.

particularly sharp. The standard management here is to smooth or remove the offending tooth and review the patient to ensure it has healed. You should beware of reviewing the patient a week later to find a significant improvement and, on that basis, discharging them. It is possible for a tooth to rub on a cancer and

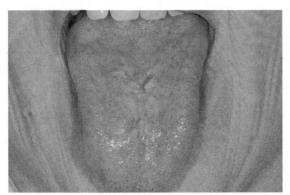

Erosive Lichen Planus on the tongue. The diagnosis is suggested by the extensive white areas. The dorsum of the tongue is low risk for cancer so in this case a biopsy was elsewhere in the mouth. Of course lateral and ventral tongue is high risk for malignancy

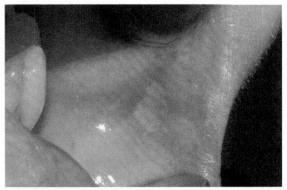

Aphthous ulcer on buccal mucosa. Note punched out appearance and typical red margin

make it more uncomfortable in the early stages. We would prefer to review the patient in two weeks, having told them the purpose is to exclude a cancer, and then carrying out a biopsy if the ulcer has not completely healed. If there is any suspicion, then biopsy on the first visit as well as attending to the tooth.

The vast majority of patients we see are reasonable human beings, but among them are a few abnormal who will harm themselves for no logical reason and produce 'factitious' ulcers. This must be at the back of our minds when seeing patients with unexplained traumatic ulcers. Those with diagnosed psychiatric disorders are generally not the problem. It is more the personality disordered neurotics who are attention seeking. A biopsy will be reported as 'non-specific ulceration'.

Erosive lichen planus

This is the most common cause of chronic oral ulceration you are likely to see. The patients are usually middle aged or elderly; most commonly, the posterior buccal mucosa and gingivae are affected but also the tongue. Look for white patches or striae on the mucosa and desquamative gingivitis. Remember, a cancer can arise from lichen planus (see the chapter on potentially malignant oral disorders).

Apthous ulcers

Are the most common acute ulcers. They are often referred by medical practitioners asking for advice. The patients are more frequently female and often young. The ulcers are usually on the movable mucosa, usually the buccal and labial areas. They are shallow, have a clear red margin and are painful. Usually they are small, being 1 - 2 mm across (minor aphthae), but

occasionally they may be much larger and deeper (major aphthae). The term herpetiform ulceration is used when they occur in large numbers which coalesce to form large lesions; this is rare. Occasionally other systemic disorders may be responsible for identical ulcers such as cytomegalovirus infection, which is associated with immune deficiency (particularly AIDS), Behçet's syndrome, cyclic neutropenia and coeliac disease. Minor aphthae are recurrent and occur in episodes which sometimes exhibit prodromal burning or tingling symptoms. The cause is unclear, but they are associated with stress and smoking is thought to be a risk factor.

Episodes of aphthous ulceration usually disappear with time and the patient should be reassured of this. In the meantime, they may be helped by topical pastes containing liquid paraffin and gelatin, which form a barrier, and benzydamine mouthwash, which is slightly anaesthetic. Topical steroids may help, particularly if applied in a prodromal phase, such as hydrocortisone pellets, triamcinolone paste or beclomethasone applied from an asthma inhaler. In severe cases, such as herpetiform ulceration, a topical tetracycline or chlorhexidine mouthwash may be helpful in reducing secondary infection, which contributes to pain.

Herpetic gingivo-stomatitis

We have listed primary in the 'less common' category of oral ulceration. It is, of course, quite common but unlikely to be seen in an oral and maxillofacial department as it is acute. It usually occurs in very young children and marks their first contact with the herpes simplex virus type 1. It remains dormant throughout life and can be reactivated later to produce herpes labialis (cold sores). Where the young child is affected, symptoms are usually very short and mild and are undiagnosed. However, if the

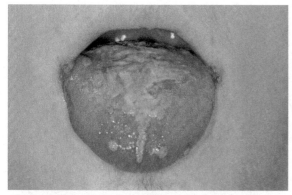

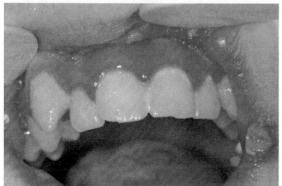

Primary herpetic gingivo stomatitis. Top: note the discreet ulcers on the anterior tongue where the vesicles have burst, behind they have coalesced producing a mass of foul slough. Bottom: the gingivae are swollen and red. This is unlikely to be referred to OMFS, this child attended the orthodontist for assessment and he asked us to see as he didn't know what it was

first contact with the virus is later, and particularly in an adult, they may be quite severe and in the worst cases, hospital admission may be necessary for supportive intravenous fluids if they cannot swallow. All the oral and pharyngeal mucosa may be affected with vesicles which rupture to form shallow painful ulcers with a red margin. The gingiva are red and swollen and the vermillion of the lip is affected. The ulcers usually coalesce to form larger ulcerated areas. There may be a prodromal phase when the patient has a tingling and burning in the mucosa; they may have a mild fever and nausea with cervical lymphadenopathy. Aciclovir may be helpful if applied early in the prodromal phase, but the condition is unlikely to be diagnosed early enough and management is 'supportive'. Herpes simplex virus type 2 is the sexually transmitted version; the lesions are similar to type 1.

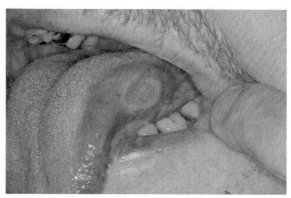

A nicorandil induced ulcer. It was smooth and flat on palpation and very painful. Differential diagnosis included cancer and trauma from the teeth. Biopsy was reported as 'non specific ulcer'

Reactivation of the herpes varicella-zoster virus, which has remained dormant in the trigeminal nucleus after the initial exposure as chickenpox, will cause eruptions of vesicles in the mouth and on the face and is known as shingles. This occurs mostly in the elderly and/or immunosuppression. It is painful and is discussed in our chapter on facial pain.

Medication induced ulcers

These are most common with nicorandil and methotrexate. A biopsy will report 'non-specific ulceration'.

Less common causes of ulceration

Acute ulcerative gingivitis has become rare in recent years, but you may see a patient referred from a primary care physician for diagnosis. There will be severe gingival inflammation, which is exacerbated by the lack of tooth brushing consequent upon the pain and bleeding. There will be ulceration of the inter-dental papillae and an unpleasant smell. The classic management in this acute state is metronidazole, but this will be unnecessary if the patient has gentle scaling from a dentist and has started gentle oral hygiene measures and chlorhexidine mouthwash.

You may see a patient with erythema multiforme. The diagnosis is easy for those who have seen cases before as the appearance is so typical. Red lesions occur on the oral and pharyngeal mucosa, which form into bullae which rupture forming large areas of painful irregular ulceration. The vermillion of the lip and skin may be involved where you may see the concentric red rings that become bullae and are known as 'target lesions'. The ulcerated areas form a horrible smelly crust with haemorrhagic areas. This is all very painful and the patient may need hospital admission for

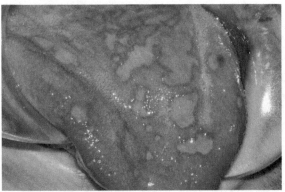

Erythema multiforme. This young man was admitted to hospital by the ENT surgeons with extensive oral and oro-pharyngeal lesions preventing swallowing. We made the diagnosis by the typical appearance of his tongue and crusted heamorrhagic ulcers of his lips extending onto the peri-oral skin. There were no predisposing illness or medication. He stayed in hospital for 5 days receiving IV fluids while unable to swallow and recovered in 2 weeks with no further recurrence

supportive intra-venous fluids if they cannot swallow. The cause is unknown but thought to be immune mediated and may be preceded by herpes simplex or some other infection or by medication, but usually no specific cause is found. Lesions usually start over a period of about a week and take several weeks to settle completely. It has been known to recur, but usually it settles completely. In severe cases, it can become Stevens-Johnson syndrome with ocular and genital involvement. This can occasionally be life threatening. Management is supportive; aciclovir may be used if herpes can be implicated and steroids have been used, but the evidence of their helping is lacking.

You are unlikely to see <u>mucous membrane pemphigoid,</u> but it is important to diagnose it and distinguish it from the much nastier pemphigus vulgaris, which also may present with similar lesions in the mouth and may be life threatening. Mucous membrane pemphigoid is usually seen in elderly females who produce red areas on the oral mucosa with bullae, which may be seen intact before rupturing, leading to an uncomfortable erosion. The lesions are not usually widespread and don't affect the skin, but they can affect the mucous membrane of the eye, leading to loss of vision. This is a different condition to bullous pemphigoid, which affects the skin primarily and rarely the mucosa.

The bullae of mucous membrane pemphigoid are sub-epithelial. The fluid forms between the epithelium

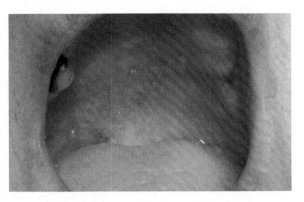

Pemphigus. The bullae on the junction of the hard and soft palate are breaking down to form ulcers with loose pieces of thin partial thickness mucosa visible. There were extensive lesions on the buccal mucosa. The patient was referred to the dermatologist and treated with immunosuppressive medication

and the connective tissue beneath. During the examination, you may test for Nikolsky's sign which involves wiping an unaffected area which produces an intact bulla. Diagnosis is by biopsy, of preferably an intact bullae, for immunofluorescence, which should show autoantibody and complement attached to the basement membrane of the epithelium. Management is usually only supportive as it usually goes away. However, topical steroids may be used on ruptured bullae or dapsone may be used, an antibiotic which has anti-inflammatory properties and is used by dermatologists for other conditions. An ophthalmic surgeon should examine the eyes.

<u>Pemphigus vulgaris</u> is more uncommon but frequently presents in the mouth. It is also autoimmune and can be fatal, so early diagnosis and referral to a dermatologist is essential. This also gives a positive Nikolsky's sign, but the mucosa tends to fragment as the bullae are intra-epithelial, i.e. within the epithelium rather than below it. Diagnosis is again by biopsy and immunofluorescence. Management is by immunosuppression.

Sometimes, chronic ulceration of the mouth may be very severe and debilitating, even compromising adequate nutrition. In this circumstance, it may justify immunosuppression with such medication as azathioprine, systemic steroids, colchicine or thalidomide. These patients are best managed in co-operation with, or exclusively by, a dermatologist who will be experienced in using these drugs, their doses and side effects; some Oral and Maxillofacial Surgeons have joint clinics with their dermatology colleagues for this purpose.

40. **Introduction to the Management of Mouth Cancer**

You should seize the opportunity to see cases of mouth cancer while in an OMFS department. See and feel the lesions, take histories from the patients and observe their treatment; this will help develop your suspicion of unusual conditions in the mouth. When practising any form of clinical dentistry a familiarity with cancer can only help with recognition and early diagnosis. You will probably be involved in taking biopsies and assisting at surgery, some of which can be quite lengthy. You should not be involved in making decisions about patient treatment. However, you may however be called by the nurses if a patient has an actual or perceived problem. You should always pass on the concern to someone more senior, usually the specialist registrar or consultant. In well run departments, post-op cancer patients will be visited by a consultant or specialist registrar at least daily until they are fit enough to go home and usually twice a day in the first few days.

The MDT

Mouth cancer will be managed, along with other cancers of the upper aero-digestive tract, by the 'Head and Neck' Oncology Multidisciplinary Team (MDT). This will have core members who will include OMFS surgeons, ENT surgeons, clinical oncologists, radiologist, pathologist and a specialist head and neck oncology nurse; there may also be a plastic surgeon. There will also be non-core members of the team who will consist of ward nurses, Macmillan nurses, who are specialists in cancer care out of the hospital, speech and language therapists who are specialists in problems of speech and swallowing, as well as dietician,

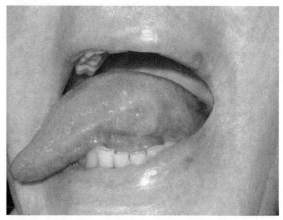

Infiltrating squamous cancer floor of the tongue. It was sore and starting to get painful.

physiotherapist, restorative dentist and dental hygienist.

Mouth cancer behaviour

Each individual mouth cancer has its own (abnormal) genetic make-up and hence its own personality. Some behave themselves when treated, but others have decided at the outset they are going to be awkward and continue to grow whatever we throw at them. It is not unusual for cancers of the tongue, especially, to erupt around the margins of a surgical resection, even though the histopathology suggests an adequate surgical margin, and then to be only temporarily impeded by post-operative radiotherapy.

Most oral cancers are managed initially by surgery, which is usually followed by radiotherapy depending on the stage and clearance at the resection margins. Large tumours may receive chemotherapy and radiotherapy before surgery to shrink them.

Following treatment, if the patient gets recurrent disease, it usually becomes apparent within the first year after diagnosis. Most remaining failures manifest themselves between one and two years and it is unusual for patients to get recurrent disease after two years. Patients who have had head and neck cancer are at increased risk of getting a second primary, particularly if they continue to smoke. The more unusual tumour may behave differently; for example, some muco-epidermoid cancers can behave very well and adenocystic cancers have a nearly 100% five-year survival rate but tend to recur much later so that the 15 year survival is low. Oro-pharyngeal squamous

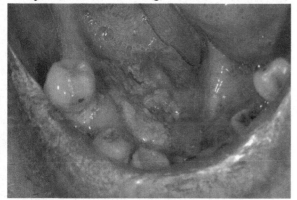

Squamous cancer floor of the mouth. Patient was alerted to it by pain; however when small the cancers will be painless. Patient was a heavy smoker and drinker of sprits; he also had an inoperable cancer of the oesophagus.

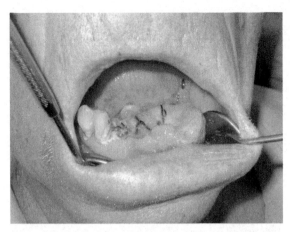

Large squamous carcinoma of the lower alveolus at presentation. The GP had treated it with mouthwashes and the dentist with antibiotics. When this didn't work he took the teeth out, hence the black silk sutures. By the time the patient was seen in hospital the tumour was deeply infiltrating into the mandible. While in hospital you must see as many cancers as possible so that you may recognise them, but any lesion you don't recognise must be treated with suspicion.

cancers related to human papillomavirus infection tend to occur in younger patients and have an overall better prognosis than other squamous carcinomas of the oral cavity.

Our cancer patients are more elderly and they are more likely to have co-existing systemic disease than most other OMFS patients and they are more likely to suffer complications of their treatment. In addition, their surgery is usually more complicated. We will therefore present a short explanation of surgical management of a typical patient with a mouth cancer requiring ablative surgery and reconstruction.

Part of the pre-operative assessment will include scanning, either CT or MRI scans, or both. If the tumour is in the maxilla, or elsewhere is extensive, then a CT scan will be requested to demonstrate the extent of bone invasion. A CT of the chest is mandatory to exclude metastatic disease in the chest.

Neck involvement

A main concern about all cancers will be the spread to the lymphatic drainage of the neck. An MRI scan can be helpful in diagnosis of cancerous infiltration of neck nodes. If enlarged or suspicious nodes are identified by palpation or on the scan, then an ultrasound-guided fine needle aspirate can be examined by a cytologist to determine whether there are metastatic cells present. An MRI will also help to

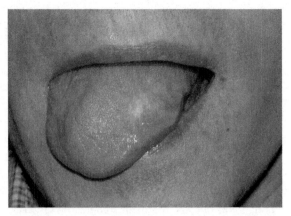

A happier tale. This patient had no symptoms & had not noticed the white patch on his tongue. His dentist referred him. A biopsy showed severe epithelial dysplasia so the whole patch was removed with CO_2 laser. Within it the pathologist found a squamous cancer penetrating 0.7 mms. A wider local excision was carried out.

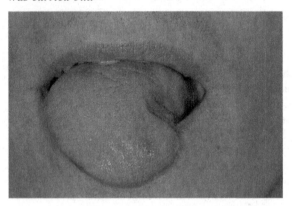

The cancer was caught early and four years later the residual tongue deformity caused no morbidity.

delineate the degree of soft tissue invasion, particularly helpful in base of tongue tumours.

Most patients with intraoral cancer will receive a neck dissection. Cancers in the tongue or anywhere in the floor of the mouth, especially large ones, have a good chance of already producing metastatic disease in the lymph nodes of the neck. This may be of an extent that it cannot be detected by clinical examination or scanning, and so nodes must be examined microscopically. Lymphatic spread tends to occur sequentially from above downwards, but with lesions on the side of the tongue, there may be skip lesions with lower nodes containing tumour while those above do not.

The radical neck dissection was described by Crile in 1904. It is the easiest neck dissection to perform and involves removal of most of the structures. It is still the operation of choice for advanced neck disease where there are several large nodes which suggest that spread outside the capsule of the node is likely. It involves removing all the structures in the neck superficial to the pre-vertebral fascia from the trapezius muscle behind to the midline of the neck anteriorly and from the clavicle inferiorly to the submandibular triangle superiorly. In addition to the nodes, the sternomastoid muscle, the omohyoid muscle, the internal jugular vein, the submandibular salivary gland and the accessory nerve in the posterior triangle of the neck are removed.

However, more frequently, we use a selective neck dissection which is permissible if there are one or two nodes without disease spread beyond their capsule. If neck disease is found to be more extensive than anticipated, then a selective neck dissection may be converted into a radical one. The advantage of the selective neck dissection is twofold. Firstly, it preserves the accessory nerve in the posterior triangle; the sacrifice of this nerve in most cases produces a shoulder syndrome due to the loss of its innovation to the trapezius muscle. The patient's shoulder droops; they cannot lift their arm above their head and attempting to do so causes the scapula to wing out. Eventually, the shoulder becomes painful, which can be helped to a certain extent by aggressive physiotherapy, but it is sacrifice of this nerve that causes the major morbidity following a radical neck dissection.

The selective neck dissection relies on the fact that oral tumours, particularly anterior ones, are unlikely to spread to the nodes of the posterior triangle. If any nodes, or suspicion thereof, are found in the posterior triangle at operation, the nerve must be sacrificed because preservation of it is not an oncologically sound procedure. The selective neck dissection also conserves the internal jugular vein; dissection of the nodes from around the vein makes the procedure fiddly and more prolonged. There are two reasons to preserve this vein. Firstly, if there is disease in both sides of the neck, sacrificing both veins will mean that the only drainage from the head will be through the vertebral veins. This will lead to severe swelling of the head, although this will probably settle with time. The most usual reason for preserving the internal jugular vein is to allow anastomosis of the venous drainage from the free flap used to reconstruct the defect caused by the cancer ablation surgery.

For a patient with a small primary tumour with no evidence of neck disease, the team will have to decide

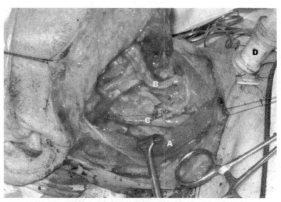

The neck completed before closing. A is the sternomastoid muscle held back by a retractor. B is the pedicle running up to the flap in the floor of the mouth. C is the internal jugular vein with the pedicle vein attached to its side. D is the tracheostomy tube.

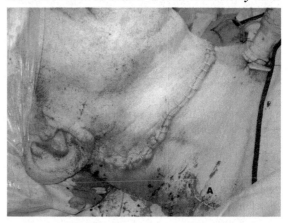

Neck closed with staples. They are quick to put in and clean and easy to remove 10 days later. This incision gives a very acceptable cosmetic result. A is a suction drain to prevent haematoma formation.

whether to watch the neck closely over a period of time for evidence neck metastases or carry out a selective neck dissection with removal of the primary tumour. But many patients will have surgery in which no cancer is detected on subsequent histological examination. A third method which is under investigation is biopsy of the sentinel node in the neck. This is the first node to receive lymphatic drainage from the tumour area. It is identified with nuclear medicine imaging by injecting the patient the day before with technetium labelled colloid, which gives off gamma rays. The node is removed via a small neck incision at the time of removal of the primary tumour and subjected to extensive histological examination. If micro-metastases are found, a selective neck dissection is carried out within a couple of weeks.

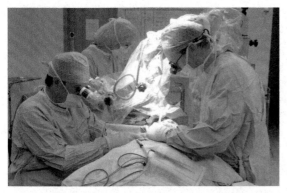

Once disconnected from the arm the flap is put into place and the radial artery is anastomosed to the lingual or facial artery and the veins to the internal jugular. The surgeon is using an operating microscope as the arteries are 1 mm diameter but the assistant is using operating loupes. This is micro-vascular surgery.

Feeding in the operative period

Most oral cancer patients receiving surgery will have a feeding tube passed into the stomach before surgery. This is to avoid them taking nutrition by mouth, which might cause a breakdown of the surgical wound margins, leading to a communication of the mouth with the neck. This complication is known as an oro-cutaneous or salivary fistula and although it usually dries up with time, this may take two or three months and in the meantime sepsis in the neck will compromise the pedicle and anastomosis of the free flap reconstruction which may die as a result. This is usually achieved with a fine bore tube passed through the abdominal skin by a radiologist using ultrasound as PUG (percutaneous ultrasound guided gastrostomy) or RIG (radiologically inserted gastrostomy). This gastrostomy tube is placed a few days before the patient is admitted to the hospital for surgery. They are trained to use the tube themselves as this can be kept in place for months and may be useful later if they are to have radiotherapy, which causes severe mucosal inflammation and hence pain during swallowing so that supplemental feeding through a tube is desirable.

The operation

The operative procedure usually starts with a tracheostomy. A cuffed tracheostomy tube is placed. This removes the inconvenience of having to operate around a nasal or oral tube which may interfere with the surgery. But more importantly, it makes the whole post-operative period safer, as the airway will not be compromised by swelling or bleeding, and, in the

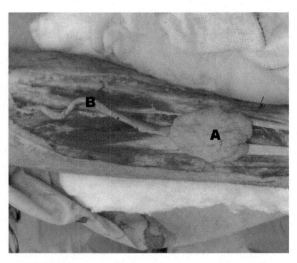

The radial forearm flap raised but not yet disconnected from the arm. It consists of skin and fascia (fascio-cutaneous). The flap A which is used to reconstruct the floor of the mouth is attached by the pedicle which consists of the radial artery and the small veins which accompany it (vena comitans). The hand is kept vital by blood supply from the ulnar artery. C is the wrist. If the mandible is to be resected a compound flap can be raised with the radius used to reconstruct the bone defect, but more commonly we use a free flap from the iliac crest or fibula from the leg.

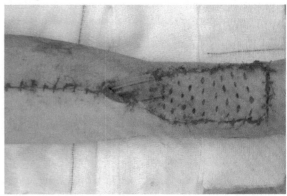

The arm donor site closed, usually with a V to Y advancement of skin, but in this case a skin graft has been used. A drain is placed to allow seepage of any bleeding. It is then bandaged.

unlikely event that the patient has to return to theatre for attention to bleeding or the flap re-anaesthetizing, will be a much simpler and safer procedure. The tracheostomy tube is usually removed three or four days post-op when we are confident that the patient can breathe through their mouth or nose and that there are no complications making re-anaesthetizing likely.

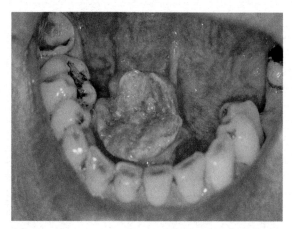

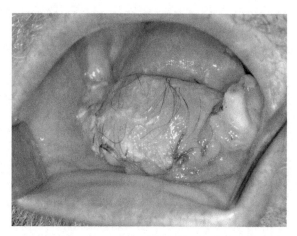

Squamous cancer in floor of mouth presented with pain. It is not involving the mandible. The treatment plan recommended to the patient by the head and neck oncology multidisciplinary team was a modified neck dissection, resection of the tumour and reconstruction with a free flap of skin and fascia taken from the forearm (radial forearm flap). This is the standard operation used in this situation. The mandible was not invaded so bone was not resected. The surgery was followed by radiotherapy. The bad teeth in the line of the radiation were removed at operation.

Following tracheostomy, the patient is prepared (prepped) with the skin wiped with disinfectant solution, usually Povidone iodine or Savlon, and draped with sterile surgical drapes. The operation proper can begin. Surgery starts with the neck dissection and then usually proceeds to resection of the primary tumour. The aim is to remove all the lymph nodes without breaching the capsules of the glands and the primary tumour with a good surgical margin (usually 1 - 2 cm). After the resection, the specimen is removed and placed on a cork board and pinned out so that it can be orientated by the pathologist who will need to dissect the specimen. He will need to know which bit he is dealing with so that he can produce an accurate report for staging. Further samples may be taken from the margins of the 'clean' resection wound and sent for histology in separate bottles for frozen sections during surgery. This is useful as an additional check, as the specimen will shrink and the pathologist's reported clearance margin may not be accurate. It will be helpful for reassurance that the tumour has been cleared (or otherwise) which will contribute to the decision on whether radiotherapy is recommended.

Following resection reconstruction is carried out, typically with a radial forearm flap, which is usually plumbed into the lingual or facial artery and internal

Three weeks later the radial forearm flap had taken nicely and was growing hair. The Vicryl sutures had not all dissolved yet. Radiotherapy was planned to start within six weeks; it stops the hair growth. At the time of writing six years had passed and the patient was alive and well.

jugular vein. Raising the flap from the forearm can be started by another maxillofacial surgeon while the resection is being completed.

Post operative care

Following surgery, the patient will go back to the ward. It will need to be a ward which is used to looking after patients with tracheostomy. The patient may be admitted to an Intensive Care Unit if they are medically unfit before surgery; often this is because of ischaemic heart or respiratory disease. If this is the case, they may be sedated and respiratory ventilation taken over by machine or the patient may breathe spontaneously assisted by CPAP (continuous positive airways pressure) or PEEP (positive end expiratory pressure). These improve airways expansion and respiratory exchange and decrease the risk of atelectasis (peripheral airway collapse).

Once back on the ward, post-operative medication will need to be reviewed and prescribed. This will now include subcutaneous enoxaparin given to prevent deep vein thrombosis. The patient should also have TED (thrombo embolic deterrent) stockings for the same purpose. Enteral feeding will be started through the gastrostomy tube; the feed will be prescribed by a dietician. The patient should now get all their fluids via the tube, and the intravenous drip may be discontinued, but the cannula should be kept for access for medication, for example, antibiotics.

On the first post-operative day, the patient will remain in bed but by the second day they should be encouraged to sit out of bed for a few hours in the

Observation:	Look for:	Significance:
Temperature	Pyrexia Temp above 38°C	Atelectasis, blood transfusion, DVT, death of donor flap, infection of chest, wound, IV lines or catheter
Blood Pressure	Decreasing BP	Inadequate fluid input, sepsis, inadequate cardiac output
Respiratory Rate	Resp. rate above 20/min	Sepsis, respiratory or cardiac insufficiency - always sinister
Local wound	Bleeding	Unless trivial should be stopped
Wound drain	Is it still draining?	Should be removed if not
Donor flap	Colour, swelling, capillary refill	Will become darker, slightly swollen with poor capillary refill if it is dying and will smell
Tracheostomy	Is the tube & surrounding skin clean, tube fully patent & secure? Check humidifier	Must be clean and patient or might block
Oximeter	Saturation close to 100, not reducing	Inadequate oxygenation
Calves	Swelling or discomfort	Signs of DVT (check prophylaxis)
Abdomen	Listen for bowel sounds	Major surgery & opiates can stop gut motility. Check before starting feeding

Post operative checks for a major cancer case. Always report any concern to the consultant or specialist registrar. Refer to chapters 14 & 34 for complications and tracheostomy

morning or afternoon. They should have their haemoglobin and blood chemistry retested on the second morning. Haemoglobin should ideally be about 10 for the best chance of flap survival. The tracheostomy should be given regular suction and humidification to prevent crusting in the tube. Suction drains should be reviewed regularly. The nurses should have recorded the amount of drainage and those draining little or nothing should be removed by day three, keeping perhaps one drain at the bottom of the neck.

The urinary catheter will have been placed to monitor the urinary output during the operation and for the first 24 hours. The nurses usually appreciate its being kept for convenience until the patient is mobilised. This should be permissible for another two or three days, but thereafter it should be removed and the patient should be encouraged to go to the bathroom or otherwise use a bottle. Prolonged retention of the catheter will pre-dispose to urinary tract infection or ulceration and possibly stenosis of the urethra. It is a

good policy to order the removal of one or two lines or tubes each morning on the ward round. The patient can then see this as a positive progression towards normality over the next few days.

It is important that the patient should have adequate pain relief. This is best achieved with an intravenous catheter attached to a syringe in a pump containing morphine, which is dispensed regularly. An additional amount may be given by the patient pressing a button if they are in pain (this is called PCA or patient controlled analgesia). These do not tend to be very painful operations and the PCA will rarely be required after a couple of days. Then regular paracetamol can be given through the gastrostomy tube and supplemented by opioid analgesics prescribed on an 'as required' basis.

A frequent problem in the post-operative period is with sleeping. A low dose of one of the more sedating tricyclic antidepressants such as dothiepin in the evening may help with this as well as having a beneficial effect on the mood later on. Usually in the first day or two after the operation, the patients are in a very positive mood, even sometimes euphoric, having discovered that they have got through the dreaded operation. They do however tend to get fed up by the end of the first week when they are getting stronger and are disconnected from all the lines and tubes except for the enteral feeding Then they are hanging around in hospital waiting for their flap to heal sufficiently for them to eat.

At about day three or four, the tracheostomy tube should be removed. The cuff in the tube should have been let down on day two and now, by placing a gloved finger over the orifice of the tube, it is possible to see if the patient can breathe round it and through the nose or mouth. If so, the tube can be removed, and a dressing placed over the wound which usually heals spontaneously. If after a few days the tracheostomy continues to blow, it should be sutured on the ward with local anaesthetic.

At a varying time, depending on the circumstances or local policy, which in our case is seven days, the margins of the reconstruction in the mouth are inspected and if all is healing well, the patient may take their first sips of water. If inspection the following morning reveals no problem with the wound margin, the patient can progress to a sloppy diet and the following day to firmer things and be discharged home. Once they can take things by mouth, enteral feeding is suspended, but the PUG tube is kept in case it is needed during radiotherapy later.

We will conclude with a few words about relatives. Occasionally they will turn up in the evening or at the weekend and want to speak to the doctor and the nurse will call you. We would strongly advise you to avoid discussion as you will not be able to provide a detailed explanation and information that they want to know about prognosis and you should always suggest that they see the consultant in charge of the case during normal working hours. Our experience has been that less experienced clinicians tend to give too optimistic an outlook based on experience of too few cases.

41. <u>The Management of Impacted Teeth</u>

An oral and maxillofacial surgery hospital department should provide you with plenty of opportunity to receive the supervised instruction necessary to become a safe dento-alveolar surgeon. Much of this work consists of removal of impacted third molars, which, for historical reasons, have been referred into hospitals. Nearly all of it could be carried out in dental practice by general dentists. Although some cases can be technically difficult, the skills to do it can be gained by a competent practitioner in a few weeks of supervised instruction and practice.

Third Molars

Mandibular third molars normally erupt between the ages of 18 and 24 years. Vertically aligned teeth will generally erupt fully but may become impacted in soft tissue if there is insufficient room in the dental arch; this may become the cause of repeated pericoronal infection. Mesially inclined teeth may gradually become vertical after eruption or impact further; they too may lead to pericoronitis, exacerbate oral hygiene and predispose to caries in the distal of the second molar; they may become carious themselves. In these cases, surgical removal is indicated. Where a patient has a part erupted mesioangular impacted third molar and poor oral hygiene with demineralisation of the distal of the second molar, then removal of the third molar should be discussed and possibly recommended to them. There is very little indication for removal of unerupted third molars.

As with all but emergency cases, the patients will initially be seen for a consultation in an outpatient clinic and an assessment carried out. Each tooth that is listed for surgery should have the reason recorded in the patient's notes and decisions should be made according to the recommendations of the National Institute for Health and Care Excellence (NICE). These are only

NICE indications for third molar removal
Unrestorable caries
Untreatable pulpal or periapical pathology
Cellulitis, abscess, osteomyelitis
Resorption of the tooth or adjacent teeth
Fracture of tooth
Cyst or tumour of the follicle
Tooth impeding surgery e.g. tumour resection or reconstruction

guidelines, so may be varied from in individual cases, but the reason must be justifiable and recorded in the patient's records. During the consultation, the patient should have the risks and benefits explained to them so that they may give informed consent for the procedure. Normally the patient should be listed for the surgical extractions to be carried out under local anaesthesia; sedation may be used for those who are apprehensive. Some surgeons carry out the surgery under general anaesthesia on a 'day-stay' basis. We think this is wasteful of resources and only rarely indicated.

When assessing the patient, consideration should be given to the angulation of the tooth. Mesioangular are the easiest to remove, followed by deeper vertical teeth with distoangular impactions, the most difficult. Obviously superficially placed teeth are easier to remove than deep. It is unusual for unerupted teeth to need removal as they infrequently lead to pathology.

When any operation is planned, there should be a clear reason (justification) written in the patient's notes and this should be done for each individual third molar. In the case of an upper tooth, which may be left unopposed by the removal of a lower, this may be a sufficient justification as removal should produce minimal side effects and complications.

Nerve Damage

Two particular complications of third molar removal need consideration, as there is some variance in opinion and practice. These are injury to the lingual and inferior alveolar nerves. Lingual nerve damage, although unusual, can be very disturbing for the patient and lead to disabling allodynia, which is worse than anaesthesia. Most injuries are temporary and usually result in paraesthesia, which gradually recovers over a couple of weeks. This is most frequently caused by placing a retractor between the lingual mucoperiosteum and bone; most frequently used is a

Third Molar Surgery Side Effects Warnings
Pain
Discomfort on eating
Swelling Bleeding
Bruising
Complications Warnings
Infection - pain
Numbness or tingling of lip or tongue with small risk of permanence
Tingling of lip

Haworth's retractor. If this instrument is used to protect the nerve from a rotating bur, it will be inadequate. A surgeon who removes lingual bone before elevating the tooth should not rely only on this retractor. Alternatively, buccal bone can be removed and the tooth split to avoid the necessity of removing disto-lingual bone.

However, many surgeons have removed third molars for years without causing damage to the nerve and have relied on their knowledge of the anatomy to avoid the nerve completely; if this technique is to be used, then the placement of a lingual retractor, so that the area of operation can be adequately visualised, is desirable. Many of the nerve injuries have been caused simply by placement of a retractor. This is principally due to inexperienced surgeons attempting to lift a flap too far forward; it is easier to lift the periosteum from the bone starting in the region of the bottom of the ascending ramus of the mandible. Cutting the tooth up from an entirely buccal approach will avoid the problem, but will usually take longer and be more uncomfortable for the patient.

The worse scenario is that if the bur injures the nerve directly, the surgeon is unlikely to know this has happened until it is realised that sensation has not recovered several weeks after surgery. In this case, the severed nerve will have retracted. If sensation is still abnormal, the nerve may be surgically explored, scar tissue removed, and an attempt made to suture the ends of the damaged nerve together. Results from this are disappointing but may be better than nothing; an attempt should be considered if the nerve has not recovered after 3 months.

Third molar roots may, occasionally, be intimately related to the inferior dental nerve and cause compression of the nerve during surgery. A close relationship between the tooth roots to the nerve can usually be predicted from a digital orthopantomograph X-ray image. Where there is doubt, a more accurate

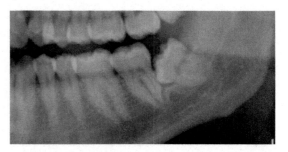

The tooth is inclined mesially and has been causing recurrent pericoronitis. The roots are close to the ID canal. Mesio-angular teeth are usually easier to remove than disto-angular or even many vertical teeth.

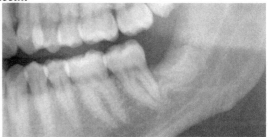

A coronectomy has been carried out on this tooth with the root close to the ID canal. Coronectomy makes the surgery easier and quicker for the patient. The remaining root often migrates upwards but needs subsequent removal infrequently. Sometimes the procedure fails when a conical root comes out completely when not intended. It should not be done for severely carious or non vital teeth.

image may be made with a cone beam computerised tomograph scan, which will demonstrate the relationship of the roots to the inferior dental bundle.

Although a cone-beam CT scan will give a better image of the relationship to the inferior dental bundle to the tooth roots, it has not been proved that this translates into less permanent nerve damage. In order to justify the additional radiation, expense and inconvenience of this, or indeed any, investigation, it should be proved that it may influence an improvement in the patient's management. Indeed, a randomised controlled trial published in the Journal of Craniomaxillofacial Surgery [2015; 43: 2158-2167] showed that the use of a CT scan did not translate into any reduction in nerve injury or of any complications. Injury to the inferior alveolar nerve can be avoided by splitting the tooth vertically for removal or simply leaving part of the root in place during surgery (coronectomy), a technique which not only has few complications but is easily accomplished

Nomenclature

Anaesthesia:- absence of sensation

Hypoaesthesia:- diminished sensation

Paraesthesia:- abnormal sensation

Dyaesthesia:- unpleasant sensation

Hyperalgesia:- increased response to a normally painful stimulus

Allodynia:- pain response to stimulus not normally painful

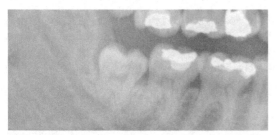

Here the distal root is dilacerated (bent) by it's close relationship to the ID canal. If the tooth is asymptomatic and there is no caries it can be retained. If there is pericoronitis or caries in the 7 or 8 it can be removed by splitting it vertically and removing the roots separately or a coronectomy carried out.

and may be less uncomfortable for the patient than removing the whole of a root with unfavourable morphology.

Damage to the inferior dental nerve does not require exploratory surgery unless it is obvious a root fragment has been pushed into the canal. Paraesthesia is usually, but not always, temporary, and allodynia is very rare. Indeed, iatrogenic injury to the inferior dental nerve occurs frequently during orthognathic surgery, as it is impossible to split the mandible sagittally without some trauma to it. Some permanent disturbance of sensation of the skin of the chin regularly occurs without causing disability.

Ectopic Canines

A frequent request from orthodontists is for surgical help with ectopic maxillary canines. Infrequently, this is to request their removal if they are very ectopic and their position and the age of the patients suggests they may cause resorption of the permanent incisors. More frequently, we are asked to uncover them surgically to facilitate their eruption or traction into the dental arch.

Much has been written about the diagnosis of their exact position with two x-rays using the parallax

X-ray signs of close root and ID bundle relation
Interruption of white lines of ID canal
Lucency across third molar root
Deviation of the canal
Narrowing of tooth root
Deflection of tooth root by canal
A better image is obtained by a CT scan but an improved outcome for the patient is yet to be proved

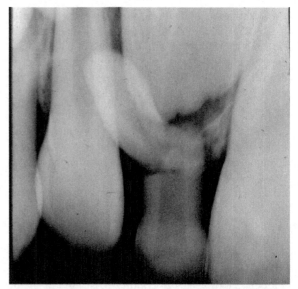

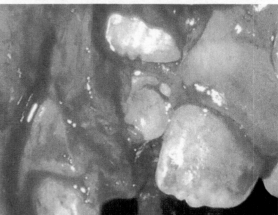

A supernumerary tooth is preventing the eruption of this permanent central incisor as seen on X-ray (top) and at operation below. Surgical removal of the supernumerary will allow the incisor to erupt. There is a lot of this minor work.

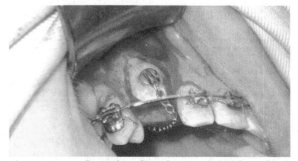

An unerupted canine has been exposed and an orthodontic bracket and chain attached with light cured acid etch seen here before wound closure.

technique, which students learn about for their examinations, or cone beam CT scans. Usually this is unnecessary, as often the tooth can be seen or palpated buccal of the dental or in the palate. If it cannot be seen or palpated, then it is usually palatal but might be high within the line of the arch. Occasionally, the apex of the tooth may be palpated in a high position buccally, while the crown is palatal. In these circumstances, the surgeon may feel more confident if the precise position has been previously revealed by a cone-beam CT scan. Similarly, when an unerupted canine is suspected of causing resorption of a maxillary incisor, a cone-beam CT scan will reveal the exact position.

Surgery can involve uncovering the tooth and suturing in a temporary pack to form a channel for eruption, the open technique. Alternatively, the tooth may be exposed and an orthodontic bracket and chain can be attached to pull the tooth in position, the closed technique. Which is used is the decision of the orthodontist who requests the treatment.

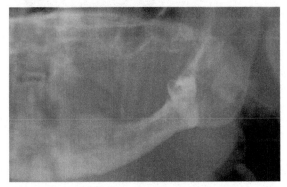

An unerupted third molar has become exposed to the mouth consequent upon alveolar bone resorption. Now causing discomfort beneath a denture and carious it needs removing

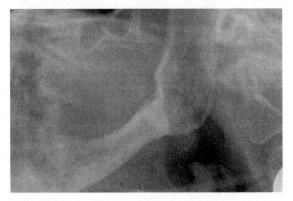

Complication. The weakened mandible has now fractured as a result of the surgery

Appendix: Eponymous Instruments in OMFS

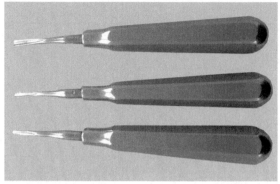

Coupland's chisels are the most used dental elevators, size 1 to 3. They can be used to split teeth that have been partly divided with a bur, and to elevate teeth and roots. Size 1 is placed between bone and tooth and rotated to move the tooth remnant into the space created with a bur. Only when some movement has been achieved should a larger size be used. They should never be used like a lever.

Douglas Charles William Coupland (1901 –1936) qualified as a dentist from Toronto in 1922. He studied exodontia at the Mayo Clinic and then practised oral surgery in Ottawa. He developed his chisels/gouges during the 1920s. They were initially produced in sets of 8 or 12, later reduced to 3.

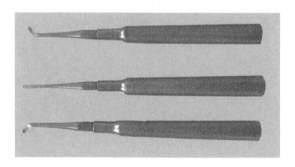

Warwick James elevators are the next most useful. There is a straight one and there are two curved, curved left and right. They are used for elevating small fragments of dental roots.

William Warwick James (1874-1965) was medically & dentally qualified, worked in dental practice as well as on the staff of the Royal Dental, the Middlesex and Great Ormond Street Hospital. He took a scientific interest in dental development, the pathology of caries and periodontal disease and wrote many books and papers, continuing well after his retirement. He fought in the First World War in France and later treated facial injuries sustained in the war. He kept all the clinical records, which resulted in a book in the 1950s. A member of the Zoological Society, he wrote about comparative anatomy of the teeth and jaws. He established a research fellowship at the Royal Dental Hospital and devised a technique for removing third molars by taking out lingual bone with a chisel. This was the forerunner of the now almost obsolete lingual split technique.

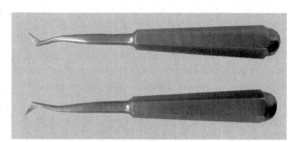

Cryer's elevators, left and right, are used to elevate the remaining single root of double rooted teeth and buccally placed upper third molars.

Matthew H Cryer (1840-1921) was born in Manchester, but emigrated to the USA when he was aged 9. He became dentally and medically qualified and was appointed Professor of Oral Surgery in Pennsylvania in 1897. He designed extraction forceps and elevators.

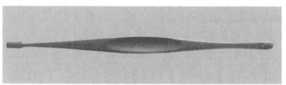

Howarth's nasal raspatory. It is used as a retractor and periosteal elevator for raising muco-periosteal flaps

Walter Goldie Howarth (1879 - 1962) was an ENT surgeon, who qualified at Cambridge in 1905 and later studied otolaryngology in Vienna & Berlin. He became the first Rhino laryngologist at St Thomas's Hospital. His instrument was devised for ENT surgery but is favoured by OMFS surgeons as well as being used in other surgical crafts.

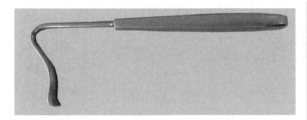

Bowdler-Henry rake retractor. Used to retract mucoperiosteal flaps during exodontia

Cyril Bowdler Henry (1893 - 1981) qualified in dentistry in 1915 and medicine in 1919. He worked in private practice in Harley Street and consulted at the Westminster and Royal Dental Hospitals. He researched into and promoted the prophylactic removal of developing third molars and diathermy in dentistry. He was one of the first surgeons in the UK to carry out osteotomies for jaw deformity. An enthusiastic supporter of dual dental and medical qualification, he donated £10,000 to the Royal College of Surgeons for a scholarship to aid young dentists or doctors to gain a second qualification.

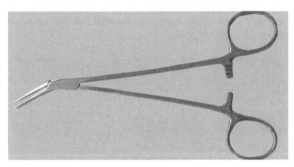

Fickling's forceps. Used to retrieve loose matter from the mouth, it has a toothed end

Ben Fickling (1909 - 2007) studied dentistry & medicine concurrently. He was one of the dentists who teamed up with plastic surgeons to treat maxillofacial war injuries. He worked with Rainsford Mowlem at Hill End Hospital, St Albans. He co-authored 'Injuries of the Jaws and Face' with Kelsey Fry and collaborated in the design of the box frame for the fixation of facial fractures. He was a founding member of the British Association of Oral Surgeons.

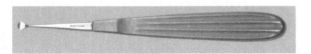

Ward's periosteal elevator

Ward's third molar retractor. The blade fits under buccal muco-periosteal flap at the angle of the mouth and gives excellent exposure of the third molar area. We still use it for those occasions when wisdom teeth are removed under anaesthetic, for mandibular osteotomies and when plating fractures at the angle.

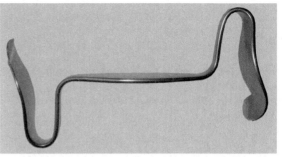

Sir Terence Ward (1906 - 1991) started his career in dentistry as apprentice to a dental mechanic and progressed via degrees in dentistry and medicine to become a founding member of the Faculty of Dental Surgery of the Royal College of Surgeons of England (and later its Dean) and the first President of the British Association of Oral Surgeons. During the Second World War he became involved at East Grinstead in treating facial injuries of RAF crew, with Sir Archibald McIndoe, and later he was appointed as the head of the OMFS service where he established a department which has trained many OMFS Surgeons.

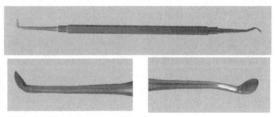

Mitchell's trimmer. Used as a curette

William Mitchell (1854-1914) trained in Michigan before moving to London, where he became a General Dental Practitioner. Mitchell invented many instruments but none as popular as his 'trimmer' which has many uses but which was probably intended to trim the cemento-enamel junction after crown preparation. (Dattani A. & Hayes S. J. Br. Dent. J. 2015; 219: 459-461)

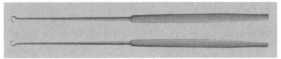

Gillies's skin hooks. Used as a pair to approximate the edges of a skin wound whilst suturing

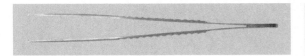

Gillies's forceps. Used to approximate wound ends while suturing. There is a toothed version which grips firmly and non-toothed version which is kinder to the tissues.

Sir Harold Gillies (1882 - 1960) was a New Zealander. He was trained as an otolarygngologist but developed many techniques for plastic surgery. In France during the First World War he worked with a dentist who was treating jaw injuries, and was inspired by the work. Eventually in England, he developed the specialist facial injury unit at Queens Hospital, Sidcup. He had a large private practice between the two world wars, but during the second, he continued his treatment of injuries at Rooksdown House, Basingstoke. There are many techniques and instruments associated with Gillies' name and he is widely considered to be the father of British plastic surgery.

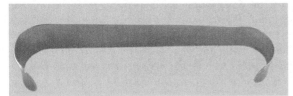

Kilner's Cheek retractor.

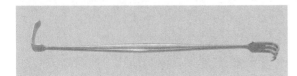

Kilner's 'Cats paw' retractor.

Thomas Pomfret Kilner (1890-1964) was one of the four original plastic surgeons who developed hospital departments, in his case at the Queen Mary Hospital Roehampton, to treat facial injuries sustained in the two world wars (The others were Gillies, McIndoe & Rainsford Mowlem). Kilner consulted at many hospitals around London and wrote about cleft lip and palate deformity and war injuries. He became a professor of plastic surgery at Oxford and was twice President of the British Association of Plastic Surgeons. He designed several surgical instruments which bear his name.

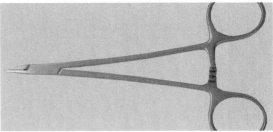

Crile-Wood needle holders. For suturing

George Washington Crile (1864 - 1943) was in the premier league of innovative surgeons. He practised in Cleveland, Ohio. He took a special interest in conditions of the head and neck and undertook thousands of operations for goitre. He travelled widely, lecturing about his techniques. He published many articles and designed many instruments. His main legacy for OMFS Surgeons was that he observed that when malignant lymph glands were individually removed from the neck, recurrent disease and death were inevitable. He developed the neck dissection in which he removed all the glands 'en bloc' after clamping the carotid artery; this often resulted in a cure. Now, over 100 years later, we routinely carry out a modification of his operation and afterwards sew up with his needle holders.

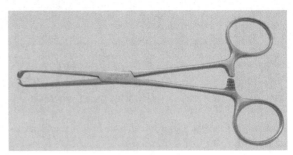

Allis forceps. Used to hold soft tissues, usually under some tension, while being removed.

Oscar Huntington Allis (1836 - 1921) practised orthopaedic surgery in Philadelphia. His chief specialism was trauma. He is known for Allis's sign in fractured neck of femur, for his splint, his dissector and his forceps, which were originally designed to retract the peritoneum.

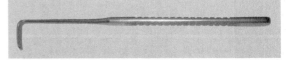

Langenbeck retractor. Available in several sizes, it is used to retract the edges of a wound while dissecting beneath.

Bernard Rudolf Konrad Von Langenbeck (1810 - 1887) was a Professor of Surgery in Berlin. He was widely known for his technique of sub-periosteal dissection for cleft palates. He discovered the yeast that we know now as candida albicans.

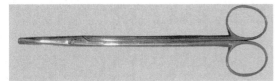

McIndoe scissors. Larger scissors for dissecting soft tissues.

Sir Archibald McIndoe (1900 - 1960) moved to England from his native New Zealand in 1930, where he joined his cousin Harold Gillies in private practice. After a spell with the American Royal College of Surgeons, he became consultant plastic surgeon for the Royal Air Force just before the Second World War. As war broke out, McIndoe moved to the newly rebuilt Queen Victoria Hospital, East Grinstead, subsequently forming the Centre for Plastic and Jaw Injuries. There he treated many burns and facial injuries where he was an innovator and teacher. He was a founding member of the British Association of Plastic Surgeons and later President. He was knighted in 1947 and became President of the Royal College of Surgeons in 1958.

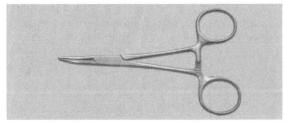

Spencer Wells forceps. Used for feeding wires between teeth, they were designed as artery clamps.

Sir Thomas Spencer Wells (1818 - 1897) was a pioneering gynaecologist at the Samaritan Free Hospital for Women and Children in London. He established ovariotomy, was a champion for public health and a rival of Lawson Tait; he became President of the Royal College of Surgeons.

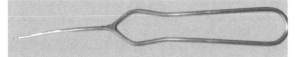

Kelsey Fry bone awl. Used to pass wires through soft tissues & around bone, usually mandible. The wire is initially fed through the hole near the tip.

Sir William Kelsey Fry (1889 - 1963) obtained dental and medical qualifications and worked during the First World War with Gillies at Queen Mary Hospital, Sidcup. Between the world wars, he worked at Guy's and during the second war at East Grinstead. Following his retirement from Guy's in 1949, he moved to the Institute of Dental Surgery as consultant in oral surgery and was subsequently Dean of the Faculty of Dental Surgery of the Royal College of Surgeons of England.

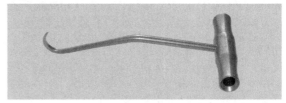

Poswillo's hook. Used to pull out a fractured malar.

David Poswillo (1927 - 2003) an OMFS surgeon, came to London from New Zealand at the age of 36 to work at the Royal College of Surgeons and subsequently at the Queen Victoria Hospital, East Grinstead. He undertook innovative research in teratology and later became head of Craniofacial Surgery at Adelaide University. He returned to London to be Professor of Oral Surgery at the Royal Dental Hospital and, when that hospital closed, Guy's. He chaired the Department of Health working party on anaesthesia in dentistry, which improved safety, and later the government committee on tobacco and health.

Rowe's Malar elevator. Used to lift a fractured malar from beneath the zygomatic arch. (Gillies's lift)

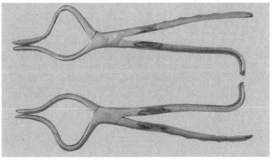

Rowe's dis-impaction forceps. Used in pairs to pull a displaced fractured maxilla forward or to move a divided maxilla forward during orthognathic surgery.

Norman Lestor Rowe (1915 - 1991) was consultant OMFS surgeon at St Mary's Roehampton and the Westminster and Eastman Dental Hospital. He was known affectionately, to his colleagues and trainees, as 'Uncle'. He initially worked in dental practice, but during WW II joined the Dental Corps, where he became involved in treating facial injuries. Later, he undertook medical and surgical training and was appointed as a consultant at Rooksdown House Basingstoke, where he worked with Gillies. After the unit moved to Roehampton, he co-wrote 'Fractures of the Facial Skeleton' with Killey, published in 1955, and later 'Maxillofacial Injuries', co-written with John Williams and published in 1985. This was, and remains, a defining text on the subject. Rowe was an innovator in the surgery of secondary cleft deformity and temporomandibular joint ankylosis. He trained many aspiring OMFS surgeons and gained wide respect and influence in the management roles he undertook. He was a defining influence on the development of OMFS as practised in the UK.

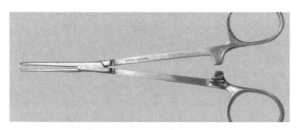

Kocher's forceps. These have interlocking terminal teeth and were designed to be used as arterial clamps. We use them as bone holding forceps.

Emil Theodor Kocher (1841 - 1917) was a German Professor of Surgery in Berne. He introduced a submandibular approach for removing cancer of the tongue. He developed several surgical instruments and was awarded the Nobel Prize for surgery in 1911.

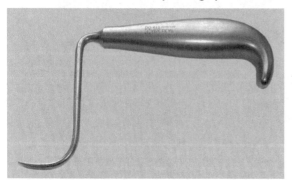

Tessier mobilizer. Used in pairs to pull forward the maxilla which has been divided.

Paul Tessier (1917 -2008) is regarded as the founder of Cranio-Facial surgery. He developed early interests in cleft lip & palate and Dupuytren's contracture but subsequently became involved with plastic surgery and burns, as well as ophthalmology. He used bone grafts to stabilise mid-facial osteotomies for severe facial deformities, an innovation which decreased relapse.

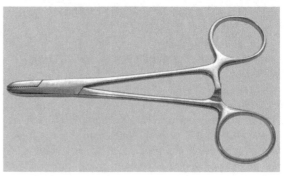

Lawson Tait forceps. Used for tightening wires, they were designed for soft tissues.

Robert Lawson Tait (1845 - 1899) was born and educated in Scotland. He practised gynaecology in Birmingham and wrote his textbook 'Diseases of Women' in 1877, as well as many other books and papers. He was a controversial figure and, for a time, was the most famous surgeon of his day. He was visited by surgeons from Europe and the USA and travelled to Canada to teach. He was a founding member and President of the British Gynaecology Society.

Acknowledgements

Oral and maxillofacial surgery like all hospital medicine and nursing has become more complicated and specialised, so it has become more difficult for authors to keep up to date with every aspect of the subjects they have written about. We have therefore become more reliant on advice and help from our colleagues who are friends.

The following have helped us with their advice or by reading our initial texts and pointing out errors and omissions and suggested changes:

Richard Thornton, consultant anaesthetist - Anaesthesia & cardiovascular assessment; Nayeem Ali, consultant OMFS Surgeon - Impacted teeth & orthognathic surgery; The late Martin Clark, consultant OMFS surgeon - Facial skin cancer; Tom Sheehan, consultant oncologist - Radiotherapy & chemotherapy; Rob Scott, consultant anaesthetist, - Fibre-optic intubation; Malcolm Read, consultant Head & Neck Pathologist - Histopathology; Graham Griffiths, consultant chemical pathologist - Blood tests; Elaine Purbrick, registered general nurse - Resuscitation, venepuncture, cross infection control; Amanda Syson, Registered General Nurses - Scrubbing and gowning; Andrew Sidebottom, consultant OMFS surgeon, - Temporomandibular Joint; Mital Patel, - consultant restorative dentist - Dental Trauma.

For advice quoted in chapter 2 - Ohsun Kwon, Sanford Grosman, Emily Illingworth, Preeya Samani, Julia Sidon, and Sara Chapman, dental core trainees and Sanaa Al Raisi, clinical fellow in OMFS.

Printed in Great Britain
by Amazon

18937245R00099